MRCOG
Oral Assessment Exam

Commissioning Editor: Ellen Green
Project Development Manager: Siân Jarman
Project Manager: Frances Affleck
Designer: Erik Bigland

MRCOG Oral Assessment Exam

Edited by

Khaldoun W. Sharif MBBCh (Hons), MRCOG, MFFP, MD

Consultant Obstetrician and Gynaecologist,
Director of Assisted Conception Services,
Birmingham Women's Hospital;
Honorary Senior Lecturer in Obstetrics and Gynaecology,
Medical School,
The University of Birmingham,
Birmingham, UK

W.B. SAUNDERS

EDINBURGH • LONDON • NEW YORK • PHILADELPHIA • ST LOUIS • SYDNEY • TORONTO 2002

WB SAUNDERS
An imprint of Harcourt Publishers Limited

© Harcourt Publishers Limited 2002

 is a registered trademark of Harcourt Publishers Limited

The right of Khaldoun W. Sharif to be identified as editor of this work has been asserted by him in accordance with the Copyright, Designs and Patents Act 1988

All rights reserved. No part of this publication may be reproduced, stored in a retrieval system, or transmitted in any form or by any means, electronic, mechanical, photocopying, recording or otherwise, without either the prior permission of the publishers (Harcourt Publishers Limited, Harcourt Place, 32 Jamestown Road, London NW1 7BY), or a licence permitting restricted copying in the United Kingdom issued by the Copyright Licensing Agency, 90 Tottenham Court Road, London W1P 0LP.

First published 2002

ISBN 0-7020-2593-3

British Library Cataloguing in Publication Data
A catalogue record for this book is available from the British Library

Library of Congress Cataloging in Publication Data
A catalog record for this book is available from the Library of Congress

Note
Medical knowledge is constantly changing. As new information becomes available, changes in treatment, procedures, equipment and the use of drugs become necessary. The editor and the publishers have taken care to ensure that the information given in this text is accurate and up to date. However, readers are strongly advised to confirm that the information, especially with regard to drug usage, complies with the latest legislation and standards of practice.

The publisher's policy is to use paper manufactured from sustainable fores

Printed in China

PREFACE

Obtaining the Membership of the Royal College of Obstetricians and Gynaecologists (MRCOG) is an essential step towards becoming a specialist in obstetrics and gynaecology in the United Kingdom and in many other countries. The Part 2 MRCOG examination has changed considerably in recent years, almost beyond recognition. Perhaps the most significant change has been the introduction of the new 'oral assessment examination'. This has replaced the traditional clinical and oral examinations which had been used in the MRCOG examination since its inception. For many candidates, the Part 2 MRCOG will be their first encounter with this new style of examination, leading to a disproportionate level of anxiety. This tends to adversely affect performance and therefore chance of success. All this is avoidable by familiarizing yourself with the oral assessment examination system: understanding what types of questions are asked, how to prepare for them and how to answer them — this is the aim of this book.

My task in writing this book has been made much easier and more enjoyable by the invaluable help I have received from my contributors, who are active clinicians at the forefront of busy clinical practice and research. Many of them are senior examiners. More importantly, they are all experienced teachers at MRCOG courses.

The advice and examples given in this book are born out of extensive experience in running MRCOG courses in the UK and abroad over a number of years. The effects that these courses have had on candidates' familiarity with the examination system, the transformation in exam performance, and their very high success rates have been remarkable. In fact, the idea for this book was suggested by a group of candidates who successfully completed one of our courses and went on to pass the MRCOG. To them, and to all the other trainees who I have been privileged to teach, I dedicate this book.

Birmingham 2001 K.W.S.

This book is dedicated to the memory of my father

CONTENTS

CONTRIBUTORS

M Afnan
Consultant Obstetrician and Gynaecologist, Birmingham Women's Hospital, Birmingham, UK

M Al-Naim
Consultant Obstetrician and Gynaecologist, Department of Obstetrics and Gynaecology, Riyadh Armed Forces Hospital, Riyadh, Kingdom of Saudi Arabia

H Al-Sawadi
Specialist Obstetrician and Gynaecologist, Department of Obstetrics and Gynaecology, Riyadh Armed Forces Hospital, Riyadh, Kingdom of Saudi Arabia

H Ba'aqeel
Consultant and Chairman of the Department of Obstetrics and Gynaecology, National Guard Health Affairs, King Khalid Hospital, Jeddah, Kingdom of Saudi Arabia

A El-Mardi
Senior Registrar in Obstetrics and Gynaecology, Burton General Hospital, Burton upon Trent, UK

H Gee
Consultant Obstetrician and Gynaecologist, Training Programme Director, Birmingham Women's Hospital, Birmingham, UK

M Hassanein
Senior Registrar in Obstetrics and Gynaecology, Birmingham Women's Hospital, Birmingham, UK

Y. Khalaf
Senior Registrar in Obstetrics and Gynaecology, St. Thomas' Hospital, London, UK.

M Lewis
Consultant Anaesthetist, Birmingham Women's Hospital, Birmingham, UK

R Mesleh
Consultant Obstetrician and Gynaecologist, Department of Obstetrics and Gynaecology, Riyadh Armed Forces Hospital, Riyadh, Kingdom of Saudi Arabia

I Morgan
Consultant Neonatologist, Birmingham Women's Hospital, Birmingham, UK

D Somerset
Lecturer in Obstetrics and Gynaecology, Birmingham Women's Hospital, Birmingham, UK

T Sabbagh
Consultant Obstetrician and Gynaecologist, Department of Obstetrics and Gynaecology, Riyadh Armed Forces Hospital, Riyadh, Kingdom of Saudi Arabia

P Toozs-Hobson
Consultant Obstetrician and Urogynaecologist, Birmingham Women's Hospital, Birmingham, UK

J Weaver
Consultant Obstetrician, Birmingham Women's Hospital, Birmingham, UK

P Wier
Consultant Obstetrician and Gynaecologist, Training Programme Director, Mater Hospital, Belfast, UK

ABBREVIATIONS

ARM	Artificial rupture of the membranes
BMI	Body mass index
BPP	Biophysical profile
BSO	Bilateral salpingo-oophorectomy
BV	Bacterial vaginosis
C&S	Culture and sensitivity
CA125	Cancer antigen 125 (test)
CCT	Controlled cord traction
CESDI	Confidential Enquiries into Stillbirths and Deaths in Infancy
CPAP	Continuous positive airways pressure
CPC	Choroid plexus cyst
CRL	Crown–rump length
CRS	Congenital rubella syndrome
CS	Caesarean section
CT	Computerized tomography
CTG	Cardiotocograph
CVS	Chorionic villus sampling
EBL	Estimated blood loss
EC	Emergency contraception
ERPC	Evacuation of retained products of conception
FBC	Full blood count
FBS	Fetal blood sampling
FHR	Fetal heart rate
GA	General anaesthesia
G&S	Group and save
GIFT	Gamete intrafallopian transfer
GSI	Genuine stress incontinence
GUM	Genito-urinary medicine
HIV	Human immonodefiency virus
HRT	Hormone replacement therapy
HSG	Hysterosalpingograph
HVS	High vaginal swab
ICSI	Intra-cytoplasmic sperm injection
IMB	Intermenstrual bleeding
IPPV	Intermittent positive pressure ventilation
IUCD	Intrauterine contraceptive device
IUGR	Intrauterine growth restriction
IUI	Intrauterine insemination
IVF	In-vitro fertilization
KOH	Potassium hydroxide
MCH	Mean corpuscular haemoglobin
MCHC	Mean corpuscular haemoglobin concentration
MCUG	Micturating cysto-urethrogram
MCV	Mean corpuscular volume
MI	Myocardial infarction
MPV	Mean platelet volume
MRI	Magnetic resonance imaging

MSU	Mid-stream specimen of urine
NT	Nuchal translucency
OHSS	Ovarian hyperstimulation syndrome
PCA	Patient-controlled analgesia
PDS	Polydioxanone suture
PET	Pre-eclamptic toxaemia
PID	Pelvic inflammatory disease
PMB	Postmenopausal bleeding
PMH	Past medical history
PMS	Premenstrual syndrome
PPH	Postpartum haemorrhage
RCT	Randomized controlled trial
SCBU	Special care baby unit
SROM	Spontaneous rupture of the membranes
TAH	Total abdominal hysterectomy
TED	Thromboembolic disease
TOP	Termination of pregnancy
TV US	Transvaginal ultrasound
UDA	Urodynamic assessment
US(S)	Ultrasound (scan)
VE	Vaginal examination
WBC	White blood cells
WCC	White cell count

HOW TO USE THIS BOOK

Begin with the end in mind

You are more likely to be successful in any task in life if you remain focused on the *aim* of that task. The aim of this book is not only to give you examples of MRCOG oral assessment questions and answers, but most importantly to help you pass the oral assessment examination. A book that gives you examples of exam questions without actually increasing your chances of passing that exam is surely a waste of both time and money. We believe that if you fully understand the system of the examination — how it is conducted and marked, the types of questions asked and how to prepare for and answer each type of question — you are far more likely to benefit from practising the examples. To get the maximum benefit from this book, therefore, we strongly recommend that you read the introductory section before you attempt any of the examples. It will help you to understand the examination system and the different types of questions, enabling you to approach them more successfully. Furthermore, in the six weeks or so between receiving the results of the written examination and sitting the oral assessment examination we recommend that you read this section once every week. It should take you no more than 30 minutes of careful reading, time well-spent in order to increase your chances of achieving your aim, that of becoming a Member of the Royal College of Obstetricians and Gynaecologists.

THE PART 2 MRCOG ORAL ASSESSMENT EXAMINATION

The Part 2 MRCOG examination consists of a written part and an oral assessment part. The written part comprises a multiple choice question (MCQ) paper and two short-answer essay papers. Only candidates who pass the written part are allowed to proceed to the oral assessment part. Candidates must pass the oral assessment examination in order to become Members of the College — the mark obtained in the written part, however high, cannot compensate for a poor performance in the oral assessment. The oral assessment examination is, therefore, the final hurdle that every prospective College Member has to overcome. For many candidates, this will probably be the first time they have ever come across such an examination system. This lack of familiarity can be overcome, however, by understanding the examination system: its evolution, importance, format and scope, the types of questions asked and how to prepare for them. This is exactly what this chapter is all about.

Evolution of the oral assessment examination

From November 1998 the oral assessment examination replaced the clinical and viva (oral) examinations in the Part 2 MRCOG. Candidates had often complained that the clinical and viva exams were neither valid nor fair. A *valid* test is one that accurately measures what it sets out to measure; a *fair* test is one that provides reproducible results (i.e. different candidates, giving the same answer to the same question, should be awarded the same mark, regardless of who is examining them). The clinical and viva exams were meant to measure skill and knowledge in various clinical scenarios and subjects but, because of the limited number of examination episodes (two clinical cases and two viva sessions), their validity was limited. In addition, different candidates were examined by different examiners on different clinical cases and asked different questions. Therefore the fairness of the exam system was also in question. The absence of a structured model answer and marking system was another drawback of the old system.

The new oral assessment examination was introduced to address all these issues. It is designed to expose candidates to a greater number of examiners and topics, and consequently to reduce the effect that any one examiner has on the candidate's score. Each candidate will be tested on the same topics as his or her peers. The general outline of the model answer and the marking system are structured and predetermined by the Examination Committee in order to increase the fairness of the exam. Although you may feel more familiar with the old examination system, the new oral assessment is actually more likely to be fair and valid. It is not surprising, therefore, that the pass-rate for candidates sitting the new oral assessment examination is higher than that for those who sat the old clinical and viva exams. *The new system works in your favour.*

How important is the exam?

Candidates and examiners alike often complain that examinations are artificial — they test candidates in tasks (e.g. essay writing, MCQs) that do not form part of their normal daily clinical work. In this sense the oral assessment examination is the most fair and real part of the MRCOG examination. It tests candidates in what they have been doing for years on a day-to-day basis: taking clinical histories, talking to patients and formulating management plans. A polished performance is therefore expected and mistakes are less likely to be excused. The required standards are high but no higher than those expected from you in everyday practice.

The importance the RCOG places on the oral assessment examination is clearly illustrated in the marking system: *however high your mark in the written paper, you must pass the oral assessment examination (i.e. score at least 60 out of 100) in order to pass the Part 2 MRCOG.*

Format of the exam

The exam consists of an assessment circuit with twelve stations. Ten of these stations will be 'active', with an examiner present, and two stations will be 'preparatory' for the following station. Each station is 15 minutes long and at some stage during the examination there will be a 10-minute break for candidates and examiners to rest and use cloakroom facilities if necessary. You will be assigned a circuit on a particular examination day and a starting station, and each time the bell rings you have to move on to the next station. The total length of the examination is 3 hours 10 minutes. The format will be identical on all three days of the examination but the actual questions will be different.

There are no real patients in the exam but some active stations will have a 'role-player' in addition to the examiner. These role-players are trained actors and actresses. In the exam they take the role of a patient or a relative, depicting a particular scenario in order to assess your communication skills. In some stations, the examiner may act as the role-player.

Examiners at each station are given general instructions about the marking scheme and how many marks are to be allocated to each part of the answer. These are for guidance only and are there to ensure as much consistency in marking as possible. The examiners have the latitude to explore in depth a candidate's knowledge and understanding.

The marking system

There are ten active stations (i.e. with examiners). Each station is scored out of 10, giving a total mark of 100. The pass-mark is 60. For each station, the examiner is given guidelines on the expected content and standard of the answer, as well as a structured marking scheme. This is to encourage consistency, but does not mean that examiners will work to a set script. As mentioned earlier, they have the latitude to explore the candidate's knowledge and understanding.

Scope of the exam

You may be asked about almost anything to do with obstetrics and gynaecology. However, the expected depth of your answer and how it is assessed will vary according to the question asked. The Membership examination is aimed at obstetric and gynaecological specialist registrars in the UK and those at equivalent grades in other countries. The knowledge expected from you is therefore similar to what you are expected to know as a specialist registrar: you should know about the detailed management of common clinical problems as well as the basic management of less common conditions. In addition to your factual knowledge, the examiners will be assessing your reasoning ability and your communication skills.

General exam techniques

Your aim in the oral assessment examination is to demonstrate your knowledge, clinical skills, common sense, analytical thinking and communication skills. The following points are worth noting as you go into the examination.

Appearance

Your Examiners will *see* you before hearing your answers. If you appear like a professional, they will be more likely to perceive you as one. Tidy hair, neat clothes and clean shoes will give you a professional appearance.

Understand the question

Listen carefully and understand the question clearly. If you do not understand the question do not simply ask the examiner to repeat it — say that you do not understand the question, and the examiner will rephrase it.

Think before you speak

Many candidates are understandably anxious which tends to make them speak very quickly, often before thinking. This should be avoided at all costs, as it is very difficult to retract what you have said. *Always think before you answer.* The examiners permit and expect you to think for a couple of seconds before you answer. If you find that your mind is totally blank and you are worried about being silent, you could say something like, 'Can I please have a few seconds to gather my thoughts?'

If, on the other hand, you realise that you have said something totally wrong (probably because you said it before thinking) the only correct thing to do is to retract what you have just said. You could say something like, 'I realise that I have just said something that is wrong. It is probably exam nerves. Can I please start again?'

Answer the question you are asked

Many different types of question can be asked about the same subject. Some candidates, under stress, go off at a tangent and answer a question totally different from the one that was asked. For example, when asked how you would manage an ampullary ectopic pregnancy laparoscopically, it is not appropriate to concentrate on the use of serial serum β-hCG levels and vaginal scans in the diagnosis of ectopic pregnancy. No matter how much you dislike the question you have been asked, or think that you can do better answering a related (but different) question, you have to play the hand you are dealt and answer the question as it is.

Self-confidence

You should exhibit a self-confident attitude: appear calm; speak in a voice that is neither aggressively loud nor timidly low and at a pace that is neither too quick nor hesitantly slow; look the examiner (or the role-player) in the eye when you are speaking; and appear to believe in what you are saying. Contrary to popular belief, self-confidence is an acquired attribute which takes much practice.

Reaction to stress

As a doctor, you are subjected to stressful situations all the time. The examiners will be trying to assess your reaction to stress by asking you difficult questions to which there may be no clear answer. Remember that only good candidates are asked these questions. Also, the role-player may depict a difficult patient (e.g. by shouting at you or being aggressive). If in difficulty, reflect on your clinical practice and imagine that you are facing the same situation in a clinical context. Do in the exam what you would do in the clinic — there is no magic, just plain common sense.

Do not repeat the question

Some examiners find candidates who repeat the questions very irritating. Whether you do it out of habit, nervousness, or because you want to gain a few seconds to think, stop doing it!

Do not dig your own grave

You have to be able to justify anything you say and explain all your proposed actions. Do not mention conditions that you know very little about. The examiners might think that you are trying to lead them up that path and, in trying to help you, they may ask you about it.

Do not argue

This is time-honoured advice, but some candidates still manage to ignore it. You may think, or even know for definite, that your examiner is wrong in something he has said, but the examination is neither the time nor the place to say so.

The questions and how to prepare

You may be asked different types of questions at different stations, each requiring a different form of answer. It is very important to understand what type of question you are being asked and to know how to formulate the answer. All too often a candidate concentrates on the *subject* in question and ignores the *form* of the question. This can result in an answer very different from what the examiner had in mind.

The following are the common forms of questions asked in the oral assessment examination, together with advice on how to answer them. The examples given are MRCOG questions which have appeared in past examinations.

1. Operative questions

You may be asked to describe an operation in detail and this may include discussion about preoperative and postoperative procedures. This will usually be about common operations which you should be familiar with. This question is usually asked in the form of a clinical scenario, for example: *A primigravid woman in spontaneous labour at term has failure of progressive cervical dilatation for 6 hours in the first stage of labour. This did not respond to artificial rupture of membranes and oxytocin infusion. You have decided to perform a caesarean section. Discuss with the consultant on call (the examiner) your preoperative, intraoperative and postoperative procedures.*

The preparation for such questions should be part of your standard training. For every operation you perform, or assist in, you should be aware of the pre-, intra-, and postoperative details. You should also be able to explain these to your colleagues. If you practice in this way, this type of question in the exam should be straightforward. This illustrates a very important point: the major part of your preparation for the Part 2 MRCOG is done during the 2 to 3 years of clinical training leading up to the exam, not just in the preceding 2 to 3 months.

2. Communication and counselling skills

Your communication skills will be assessed by your interaction with a role-player depicting a particular scenario. For example, you may be told: *The role-player has had an unexplained intrapartum stillborn baby, at term, on that day. Counsel her and explain further investigations and management.* Alternatively, you may be told: *The role-player is the husband of a woman who has had an unexplained intrapartum stillborn baby, at term, 6 weeks previously. Counsel him and explain the investigations findings (which you are provided with) and further management.* Other situations might include explaining abnormal smear results or abnormal antenatal screening test results to a role-player.

These communication skills questions should cause no difficulty for candidates who have been communicating with patients and colleagues for a minimum of 4 years before sitting the Part 2 examination. However, the pressure of the examination might make you forget a few important points. These include: introducing yourself to the patient; putting her at ease; establishing appropriate eye contact with the patient (*not* the examiner); listening attentively; explaining the condition without the use of medical jargon; following verbal and non-verbal clues; pausing for the patient to ask questions and introduce new issues; and adequately explaining the intended course of action. Finally, all communications with patients should end with the question, 'Is there anything you would like to ask me?' or something similar. In such communication stations your impression on the role-players is as important as your impression on the examiners. In fact, the role-players contribute to your mark by indicating whether they have gained confidence in you during the encounter and their willingness to see you as their doctor again.

A common mistake candidates make in these stations is to look most of the time at the examiner and the not at the role-player. This is a common cause of poor performance in such stations: you should communicate with the role-player as you would communicate with a patient in your clinic. Eye contact is fundamental in face-to-face communication. Although the examiner is there, you should try to ignore his presence and concentrate only on the role-players when you are speaking to them.

3. History-taking

Your history-taking skills will be assessed in some stations: the role-player may appear as a patient presenting with a complaint, with a GP referral letter or as an emergency. This could be in either obstetrics or gynaecology, e.g. *This 24-year-old woman has vaginal discharge. Take a full history from her and explain your further management*, or *This woman is 30 weeks pregnant and is presenting with lower abdominal pain. Take a full history from her and explain your further management.*

History-taking is actually a part of your everyday work as a junior doctor, and a polished performance is expected from you in this type of question. The key to delivering such a performance is to adopt a methodical approach, starting with the history of the presenting complaint; the past obstetric, gynaecological, medical and surgical histories; the social history; and the family history. Here again, your concentration should be on the role-payer, not the examiner.

4. Management questions

This type of question is a clinical question requiring a clinical answer. You may be presented with a clinical problem or given an investigation result and asked how you would manage it, e.g. *How would you manage an 18-year-old girl presenting with primary amenorrhoea and a serum prolactin of 2200 mU/L?*

Notice that the examiner wants to know how *you* would manage these cases. Therefore, your answer must start with '*I* would . . .'. This will give the impression that you are answering from clinical experience, rather than from book knowledge alone. You should also answer along the traditional clinical lines of history, examination, investigations, etc. Your answer should be like this: 'I would take a full history and perform an adequate examination. In the history I would want to know about . . . . In the examination I would look for . . .', and so on.

There may be different management options and you will be expected to discuss the arguments for and against each option. You should also indicate which option you would choose and why. Simply just to sit on the fence is not adequate. Similarly, to choose an option because 'my consultant says so' is unacceptable. Any controversial topics discussed in the oral assessment examination will be common clinical conditions which you should have met, read about and considered during your training.

5. Surgical instruments

You may be given a piece of surgical equipment and asked to describe or assemble it. For example, in one recent examination candidates were given a cystoscope and asked to assemble it. The main part of the station was the discussion with the examiner about the uses of that instrument. Other instruments that you may be given include obstetric forceps, a ventouse, a laparoscope or a hysteroscope.

Sometimes you may be given an instrument which you have never seen before: think again. If you are still sure that you do not know what it is, then say so. The examiners know that different instruments are used in different hospitals and with your relatively limited experience at this stage you are not expected to recognize every instrument. The examiners will then try to give you clues that may help you to recognize the instrument. For example, a candidate may be given Fallope rings but, having never used them before, may not recognize them. If the candidate says so, the examiner may say that an alternative is the Filshie clip, enabling the candidate to get back on the right track. Remember that the main point of this station is the *clinical* discussion.

6. Questions about emergencies

These are a must, and almost every candidate is asked about the management of some form of emergency during the examination. For example: *How would you manage a patient with severe postpartum haemorrhage?; How would you manage a patient with eclampsia?; How would you manage a patient with shoulder dystocia?*

Your answer must be practical, precise and direct. You should also mention first things first: *the sequence of your proposed actions is of vital importance.* There is only a limited number of emergencies in obstetrics and gynaecology, and you should practise answering questions about all of them in preparation for the exam. Remember that neonatal resuscitation is an obstetric emergency — it is also a common question in the exam.

7. Clinical skills

You may be asked to demonstrate clinical skills on special dummies in the exam, such as speculum insertion, insertion of a laparoscope or cardiopulmonary resuscitation. This will be followed by a related discussion.

You have been performing all these clinical skills during your clinical work. Candidates are often very good at knowing *how* to do things. What they are not so good at, however, is knowing *why* they do them that way. For everything you do there should to be a reason. The way to practise for this type of question is to think of everything you do at work, how you do it and why you do it.

8. Audit

You may be asked to design and discuss a particular audit protocol. A typical example might be: *Design an audit protocol for induction of labour in post-term pregnancy*. This type of question will be given to you in a 'preparatory' station, where you will have 15 minutes to consider the issue and design the protocol before discussing it with the examiner at the next station.

Some candidates often confuse the terms 'research' and 'audit'. Basically, the aim of research is to find the best way to do something. Research might be used for example, to answer the question: 'Is labour induction in post-term pregnancy better than expectant management?' *Audit*, on the other hand, is aimed at finding out if the right thing (or what we believe to be the right thing) *is being done*. For example, if our policy is to induce labour at 42 weeks gestation (because we believe it to be the right thing), we can do an audit to find out if we are actually doing this. In order to do an audit of a particular practice you should decide first on a 'gold' standard with which you will compare your practice. You should then develop methods for collecting reliable information about your practice. This information is analysed and compared with the agreed gold standard. Reasons for any disparities should be explored and ways of improving practice should be discussed and implemented. The audit cycle is completed by re-auditing the same issue after a reasonable period of time.

9. Critical appraisal and discussion of a short document

You may be asked to critically appraise a short document (such as a case report, audit report, list of guidelines, patient information sheet, etc.). For example, you may be given a patient leaflet about endometriosis and asked to critically appraise it. This type of question will be given to you in a preparatory station, where you will have 15 minutes to read the document and consider its contents before discussing it with the Examiner at the following station.

The key to critical appraisal is to recognize what the document is trying to achieve, and assess whether it has done this properly. We have already discussed what an *audit* should do, and how, in the previous section. A *case report* should briefly describe an interesting case that illustrates a useful educational point, which is not within the realm of everyday knowledge or mainstream textbooks. It should also include some sort of review of previously published similar cases, with comment on how this case differs from them. *Guidelines* are systematically developed statements which assist clinicians and patients in making decisions about appropriate treatment for specific conditions. They should address a specific clinical situation, be unambiguous, and should be based on the best available evidence. *Patient information leaflets* should be clear and written in lay-person terms with no medical jargon. They should be factually accurate and include information on benefits, risks, side-effects and limitations (as appropriate). Try to critically appraise some guidelines and patient information leaflets in your hospital using these principles. You will find that using a systematic approach is a great advantage.

In appraising any document, you should assess the strength of evidence it contains, or is based on. A commonly used *classification of levels of evidence* was produced by the US Agency for Health Care Policy and Research. This divides evidence into:

Level Ia Evidence obtained from meta-analysis of randomized trials

Level Ib Evidence obtained from at least one randomized controlled trial

Level IIa Evidence obtained from at least one well-designed controlled study, without randomization

Level IIb Evidence obtained from at least one other type of well-designed quasi-experimental study

Level III Evidence obtained from well-designed non-experimental descriptive studies and case studies

Level IV Evidence obtained from expert committee reports or opinions and/or clinical experience of respected authorities

Recommendations based on evidence are also graded according to the level of evidence on which they were based. A commonly used grading system is:

Grade A Requires at least one randomized controlled trial as part of a body of literature of good overall quality and consistency addressing the specific recommendation. *(Evidence levels Ia, IIb)*

Grade B Requires the availability of well-conducted clinical studies, but no randomized clinical trials on the topic of the recommendation. (*Evidence levels IIa, IIb, III)*

Grade C Requires evidence obtained from expert committee reports or opinions and/or clinical experience of respected authorities. Indicates absence of directly applicable clinical studies of good quality. *(Evidence level IV)*

10. Clinical understanding and setting priorities

You may be given a scenario where you have a number of clinical cases with varying degrees of urgency and asked to prioritize and divide the work between yourself and a number of doctors working with you. For example, you may be shown a 'labour ward board' which contains information on a number of patients: one patient may have a prolonged second stage with an occipito-lateral position, another also has a prolonged second stage but with a direct occipito-anterior position, and a third patient needs intravenous access because she is in active labour and has had a previous caesarean section. You are told that you have with you an experienced career SHO and a GP-trainee SHO and asked how you would divide the work and why. In this situation you would see the first patient yourself and probably deliver her in theatre as a trial; send the career SHO to the second patient; and ask the GP trainee to attend to the last patient. The examiner will discuss with you the reasons behind your choices and may introduce other clinical variables to see how you would respond to them. You are faced with similar situations every day in your clinical work. The best practice is to know the reasons behind any clinical choice you make.

11. The 'set topic' question

This is usually an open question about a particular subject, and is similar to the old-style conventional oral examination. '*Tell me about hysteroscopy*' and '*Tell me about endometriosis*' are examples. The examiners are giving you an open invitation to display your knowledge about a topic which they expect you to know well.

This is a golden opportunity for you to demonstrate the breadth of your knowledge and you should deliver a polished performance. Your answer should be factual and organized, and you should not appear as if you have never thought of this subject before.

12. Eponymous questions

An eponym is the name of a disease, structure, operation or procedure derived from the name of the person who first discovered or described it. Such questions are not infrequently asked in the oral assessment examination, not as a separate station but as a part of other stations: *Who was Braxton Hicks?; Who was Kielland?; Who was Doppler?; Who was Pfannenstiel?*

These questions should never be a cause for concern, as they are almost always asked of good candidates and can only attract bonus marks. The examiners would expect you to know the association of the eponym and the person's country of origin and occupation (most, but not all, were obstetricians and gynaecologists). A collection of such eponyms (collated specifically for MRCOG candidates) has been published in Sharif and Weaver MRCOG Survival Guide, 2nd Edn. (WB Saunders, 2000).

Practice makes perfect

Having read this section, you should now be clear about the importance of the oral assessment examination in the MRCOG, the types of questions asked, and how to prepare for and answer each type. What is needed next is practice.

The rest of this book comprises 10 oral assessment examinations each containing 10 stations. Every station contains candidate's instructions, examiner's instructions, and role-player's instructions, as appropriate. The examiner's instructions outline the general points of the expected model answer, and the marks to be allocated to each item. This general outline is the skeleton on which you will put the flesh of your answer. In some questions the examiner is instructed to inquire about certain issues, and these are included in the examples. If the candidate does not mention these points, the examiner will prompt him with specific questions. The marking system we have provided aims to give you a flavour of how different points of the answer are marked.

We wish you good luck in your exam, but remember that the more you practise the 'luckier' you will become: chance, it is said, favours only the prepared.

ORAL ASSESSMENT EXAMINATION

1

STATION 1.1

Establishment of pneumoperitoneum at laparoscopy

Marks

Candidate's instructions

This is the first time that you are operating in this operating theatre. The procedure you are about to carry out is a laparoscopic sterilization. The patient is of average build, height and weight (body mass index 23). She has completed the consent form properly and is aware of the risks of the procedure. She has been given a GA and is placed in Loyd-Davis position. The bladder has been emptied and a uterine manipulator is in place.

Demonstrate how you would produce a pneumoperitoneum, and explain each step.

Equipment available:

- Veress needles
- Gas tubing with Luer connections
- Pneumoflator
- Demonstration abdomen
- Syringe.

Examiner's instructions

The marks should be allocated as follows if the candidate:

- Checks that the spring-loaded obturator is functioning correctly — no obstruction, no bends etc. **1**
- Connects gas tubing correctly; occludes the system at the tap on the Veress needle; and notes flow reduces to zero (no leaks in system) **1**
- Releases flow, notes baseline pressure in system (in air or fluid) **1**
- Elevates abdominal wall away from great vessels and inserts the needle pointing at the sacral hollow, while the patient is still in the horizontal plane (i.e. no Trendelenburg) **2**
- Aspirates using syringe — checking there is no blood or fluid; does not waggle the tip of the needle **1**

- Injects 5–10 ml of fluid and aspirates; no fluid should be aspirated (Palmer's test) **1**
- Checks gas infusion pressure increases over baseline, but remains within 0–10 mm Hg range. **1**

Question: On aspiration of the Veress needle you obtained liquid bowel content. What would you do next?

- Leave needle in situ **1**
- Proceed to laparotomy. **1**

Total mark out of 10

STATION 1.2

Ovarian carcinoma — role-play

Marks

Candidate's instructions

Mrs Smith is a 49-year-old hairdresser. She attended the accident and emergency department a fortnight ago following a fall in which she fractured her ankle. The orthopaedic house officer noted that she complained of a 'heavy dragging' sensation in her lower abdomen and of difficulty passing urine on occasion. Prior to discharge she had a pelvic ultrasound which showed a large mass arising from the pelvis, most likely to be ovarian in origin. It was multiloculated with several suspicious-looking solid areas. Her CA125 was 462 u/ml and the laboratory results on other tumour markers were not yet available. The house officer told Mrs Smith that she had an ovarian cyst.

She returned to the gynaecology clinic today for further discussion of her results. Your task is to discuss her diagnosis and further surgical management.

Examiner's instructions

Marks should be awarded as follows:

	Marks
• Introduction, the use of non-medical jargon and eye contact	3
• Correct explanation of ovarian cyst — suggestive of carcinoma but requires laparotomy to confirm diagnosis	3
• Correct explanation of the tumour marker result	3
• Correct explanation of the possible need for further medical treatment	3
• Explanation of the possible side-effects of chemotherapy	3
• Listening to the patient and inviting questions	3
• Empathy when breaking news of the possibility of cancer	3
• Doesn't rise to challenge an angry patient	3
• Apologises for the fact that the correct diagnosis was not given while an inpatient and acknowledges feelings of grief	3
• Knowledge of inherited ovarian cancer conditions and the possibility of screening daughters.	3

Total mark out of 30: divide by 3 for final mark

STATION 1.3

Epilepsy and pregnancy

Marks

Candidate's instructions

A 33-year-old known epileptic and her husband have come to see you for counselling. She is currently taking sodium valproate (Epilim) which was found to be the only drug to control her fits effectively. They would like to start a family.

Examiner's instructions

The following questions should be asked, and the marks awarded as follows:

1. ***What pre-pregnancy advice would you offer her?***
   - Continue with the drug 2
   - Take folic acid 5 mg/day for 3 months before pregnancy. 2
2. ***What is the main adverse effect of sodium valproate on the fetus?***
   - Neural tube defect (approx. 1%). 2
3. ***So what needs to be done during pregnancy?***
   - Detailed fetal ultrasound scan and maternal serum α-fetoprotein 4
   - Take folic acid 5 mg/day for first 3 months of pregnancy. 2
4. ***What may happen to her epilepsy during pregnancy?***
   - Increased drug requirements. 2
5. ***Why?***
   - Nausea and vomiting, increased blood volume, increased binding globulins. 3
6. ***Presentation and examiner's discretion.*** 3

Total mark out of 20: divide by 2 for final mark

STATION 1.4

Audit of postnatal thromboembolic prophylaxis — preparatory station

This is a preparatory station. You are asked to design an audit protocol to find out if postnatal patients at high risk of thromboembolic complications are receiving prophylactic subcutaneous heparin in your hospital. You will be asked in the next station to explain your protocol to the examiner who will discuss it with you.

STATION 1.5	
Audit of postnatal thromboembolic prophylaxis — examination station	Marks

Examiner's instructions

The candidate will present his audit protocol and the following points should be discussed, with marks awarded as follows:

	Marks
• Establishing a gold standard to measure practice against (e.g. for all CS patients)	**4**
• Collecting data on actual practice	**4**
• Analysing these data and comparing them with the gold standard	**4**
• Presenting the results with suggestions on how to improve practice	**4**
• Implementing these suggestions and re-auditing after a reasonable period.	**4**
Total mark out of 20: divide by 2 for final mark	

STATION 1.6	
Antenatal screening for Down's syndrome — role-play	Marks

Candidate's instructions

A 38-year-old woman is referred by her GP to discuss antenatal screening tests. She has had one first trimester miscarriage and is currently 8 weeks pregnant. One of her friends had a Down's syndrome baby and she is very worried about the same happening to her. She knows that there are tests that carry no risk to the baby that will tell her whether the baby is normal or not. She does not understand which one is best. Your task is to explain the tests to her and help her to come to a decision as to which test she will have.

Examiner's instructions

Marks should be awarded as follows:

- Advice should be given about the background risk of chromosomal abnormality. For example, the risk of trisomy 21 at birth is about 1 in 150 at this age. The risk of trisomy 21 at 12 weeks is about 1 in 90. **2**
- Screening procedures for the detection of trisomies 21, 18 and 13 include measurement of fetal nuchal translucency by ultrasound at 10–14 weeks gestation. **2**
- The sensitivity of fetal nuchal translucency measurement in the detection of trisomies is about 80% with a false-positive rate of 5%. **2**
- Serum biochemistry can be offered after 15 weeks gestation as a method of screening for Down's syndrome. **2**
- The sensitivity of serum biochemistry for the detection of Down's syndrome is 65% with a false-positive rate of 5%. **2**
- Screening by ultrasound at 20 weeks may detect about 50% of Down's syndrome fetuses. **2**
- No screening test can *guarantee* a normal baby. **2**
- Alternatively, invasive testing for fetal karyotyping may be offered either routinely or following the results of the above screening techniques. **2**
- Chorionic villus sampling (CVS) is appropriate from 11 weeks gestation and amniocentesis from 15 weeks. **2**

- In expert hands, the miscarriage risk attributable to first trimester CVS is 1–2% and to second trimester amniocentesis is approximately 0.5–1%. 2

Total mark out of 20: divide by 2 for final mark

STATION 1.7

Complication at caesarean section

Marks

Candidate's instructions

You are the registrar on call for the labour ward. Your consultant is the only senior person above you (there is no senior registrar). It is 2 a.m. You have had a primigravid patient in the second stage of labour for 2 hours with no progress. After discussion on the telephone with your consultant, it has been agreed that you should proceed to caesarean section. He is confident in your ability and you proceed with the operation with your SHO assisting.

The patient has an epidural anaesthetic in situ and this has been topped-up effectively for the caesarean section. You begin the operation through a Pfannenstiel incision. The baby is larger than expected and more difficult to deliver than any you have experienced before. The baby's head is impacted in the pelvis. The Syntocinon has been discontinued for 30 minutes.

The examiner is going to ask you questions on the management of this case.

Examiner's instructions

The aim of this question is to present the candidate with a scenario in which there has been some difficulty with the delivery of the head during a routine caesarean section. A lateral tear has occurred at the left margin of the transverse uterine incision, extending down to the vaginal vault. The candidate is asked to respond to your questions on the management of this case in a safe, logical and effective manner. The following questions should be asked and marked as indicated:

1. ***What measures might you take to disimpact the head?*** **4**

   - Vaginal pressure (preoperative/during section)
   - Intraoperative — manual or forceps.

2. ***The baby and placenta are successfully delivered. The pelvis is, however, full of bright-red blood and there is active haemorrhage from the operation site. What do you do?*** **4**

   - Alert anaesthetist
   - Crossmatch blood
   - Consider general anaesthetic
   - Check uterine tone

- Locate source of haemorrhage
- Deliver uterus up into wound.

3. ***You discover a left lateral-angle tear extending towards the vaginal vault, from which there is arterial haemorrhage. Blood loss is over 1000 ml. What do you do next?*** **4**

   - Inform/request help from consultant
   - Deliver uterus up to wound
   - Identify bleeder
   - Choice of suture material.

4. ***The haemorrhage has been arrested and your consultant arrives. Before you finish the section what checks do you need to carry out?*** **4**

   - Uterus empty?
   - Syntocinon infusion
   - Blood loss overall?
   - Fluid input/urine output — catheter
   - Uterine tone
   - Antibiotics?
   - Position of ureter.

5. ***What postoperative instructions do you leave and what else do you need to attend to after concluding the operation?*** **4**

   - Level of postop care — high-dependency or alternative
   - Frequency of observations
   - Correct blood replacement
   - Fluid and analgesia management
   - Talk to patient/partner
   - Baby.

Total mark out of 20: divide by 2 for final mark

STATION 1.8

Hyperprolactinaemia

Marks

Candidate's instructions

Discuss how you would manage an 18-year-old girl presenting with secondary amenorrhoea and a serum prolactin of 2200 mU/L.

Examiner's instructions

Marks should be awarded as follows:

- History (including menstrual) 2
- Drug history 1
- Exclusion of pregnancy 1
- Examination 1
- Investigations (including pituitary imaging: CT, MRI). 2

At this stage the Examiner should tell the candidate that a micro-adenoma is found.

- Further management (dopamine agonist) 2
- Presentation and examiner's discretion. 1

Total mark out of 10

STATION 1.9	
Emergency contraception	Marks

Candidate's instructions

A 25-year-old woman is requesting emergency contraception (EC). Discuss with the examiner how you will counsel this patient and the different options you are going to offer her.

Examiner's instructions

Marks should be awarded as follows:

	Marks
• Taking a history of the timing of all instances of unprotected intercourse in current cycle	1
• Past medical history (contraindications)	1
• Yuzpe method	1
• IUCD	1
• Progestogen-only method	1
• Knowledge of recent WHO data indicating that progestogen-only EC is more successful than the Yuzpe method	1
• The earlier the hormonal methods are taken, the more successful they are	1
• Advice regarding future contraception	1
• Presentation and examiner's discretion.	2
Total mark out of 10	

STATION 1.10	
Caesarean section	Marks

Candidate's instructions

A primigravid woman in spontaneous labour at term has failure of progressive cervical dilatation for 6 hours in the first stage of labour. This did not respond to artificial rupture of the membranes and oxytocin infusion. You have decided to perform a caesarean section. Discuss your preoperative, intraoperative and postoperative procedures with the examiner.

Examiner's instructions

Marks should be awarded as follows:

- Informed consent 2
- Need to inform anaesthetist and paediatrician 2
- Left-lateral tilt on operating table 2
- Bladder catheterization 2
- Thromboembolic prophylaxis 2
- Prophylactic antibiotics 2
- Operative details 4
- Postoperative observations 2
- Presentation and examiner's discretion. 2

Total mark out of 20: divide by 2 for final mark

ORAL ASSESSMENT EXAMINATION

2

STATION 2.1

Azoospermia

Marks

Candidate's instructions

A man investigated for infertility was found to have no sperm in the ejaculate. He has no sexual problems and has normal male secondary sexual characteristics. His wife has no history of significance, and was found to be ovulating and had patent tubes. *How would you manage their case?*

Examiner's instructions

The following points should be covered, and the marks awarded as follows:

- Medical and surgical history, particularly history of: chemotherapy, radiotherapy, inguinal surgery, vasectomy, orchitis, sexually transmitted illnesses — 4
- Drug history (androgens, steroids, antihypertensives, chemotherapy) — 2
- Testicular examination (small testis suggestive of testicular cause; normal size suggestive of post-testicular cause) — 2
- Investigations (repeat seminal fluid analysis, serum FSH, karyotype) — 4
- Management if post-testicular: surgical re-anastomosis; sperm aspiration/intracytoplasmic sperm injection (ICSI) — 2
- Management if testicular: (sperm aspiration/ICSI; donor insemination (DI) — 2
- Presentation and examiner's discretion. — 4

Total mark out of 20: divide by 2 for final mark

STATION 2.2

Laparoscopic sterilisation — preparatory station

Candidate's instructions

This is a preparatory station. You are provided with the following patient information leaflet. Please read it in preparation for the next station where you will be asked to critically appraise it.

Patient Information Leaflet
Laparoscopic Sterilisation

You will be having a laparoscopic sterilisation operation. This is usually done as a day case — you are admitted, have the operation and go home on the same day. The operation will be performed under general anaesthesia and involves inserting a scope through a small (1 cm) cut at the umbilicus to have a look at the fallopian tubes, where the egg and sperm normally meet. By blocking these tubes the sperm will be prevented from meeting the egg and you will not be able to get pregnant. The tubes are blocked by applying special clips to them using an instrument inserted through another small cut in the abdomen.

The operation is irreversible: once it is done it cannot be undone. However, there is a chance that it might fail and some women will get pregnant after having the operation. This happens once in every 10 000 cases. If you become pregnant after sterilisation, there is a high chance that this pregnancy could be in the tube (ectopic pregnancy). This is a serious condition that can be life-threatening and usually requires an operation to sort it out. Also, in some women the operation makes periods heavier and more frequent.

STATION 2.3

Laparoscopic sterilisation — examination station

Marks

Examiner's instructions

There are several deficiencies and inaccuracies in this information leaflet, and marks should be awarded if the candidate detects them as follows:

- There is no mention of possible operative complications (injuries, bleeding, the need for laparotomy). **4**
- The leaflet states that the operation is irreversible. This is not strictly correct (reversal success rate is about 60% for clips). Rather, it should be *considered* irreversible as irreversibility is unpredictable. The woman may know someone who has had a sterilisation successfully reversed, which would undermine her confidence in the accuracy of the leaflet. **4**
- It states that the operation may cause the periods to become heavier. This was suggested by early studies but was later found to be incorrect. **4**
- The candidate should be aware of the recent controversy about the long-term (10-year) failure rate for some methods (up to 35 per 1000). This has not yet been assessed for Filshie clips. **4**
- Presentation and examiner's discretion. **4**

Total mark out of 20: divide by 2 for final mark

STATION 2.4	
Antepartum haemorrhage	Marks

Candidate's instructions

Discuss how you would manage a primigravid woman at 31 weeks gestation presenting with minimal vaginal bleeding.

Examiner's instructions

Marks should be awarded as follows:

	Marks
• History	**3**
• Examination	
— general	**2**
— abdominal	**2**
— pelvic (speculum, no digital VE before excluding placenta praevia)	**2**
• Maternal investigations (FBC, blood group, USS)	**3**
• Fetal investigations (CTG and USS).	**2**

At this stage the Examiner should tell the candidate that a major placenta praevia is found

• Further management/Anti-D	**2**
• Presentation and examiner's discretion.	**4**

Total mark out of 20: divide by 2 for final mark

STATION 2.5

Latex allergy

Marks

Candidate's instructions

A nurse has a history of latex allergy and is scheduled to undergo an abdominal hysterectomy. *What precautions would you and your colleagues take to avoid precipitating an anaphylactic reaction to latex?*

Examiner's instructions

The answer should contain the following points, and marks should be allocated accordingly:

- Inform the theatre manager who should disseminate the knowledge to the appropriate staff. 1
- Inform the anaesthetist responsible for the case. 1
- The patient should be scheduled to be first on the list in a theatre that has preferably not been used overnight. Latex allergens are airborne and should be at a minimal level under these circumstances. 1
- Ensure the availability of a latex-free trolley/cart and emergency drugs for the treatment of an anaphylactic reaction should it occur. 2
- Avoid the use of latex-containing material — particularly latex gloves — and cover latex-containing surfaces. 1
- Use latex-free anaesthetic circuits, face masks and monitoring equipment. 1
- Draw up drugs in latex-free syringes and avoid drawing up or administering drugs through latex bungs — place a three-way tap in the system. 1
- Presentation and examiner's discretion. 2

Total mark out of 10

STATION 2.6

Neonatal death — role-play

Candidate's instructions

You are the obstetric consultant of a patient whose newborn baby died 36 hours previously. You are going to see the patient and her husband to discuss the death of their baby. At the time of the death you were out of the country and the case was handled by your registrar and the paediatric staff.

The details you have been given by your staff are as follows:

Mrs Dawson was a 34-year old woman in her first pregnancy who presented at 41 weeks, in labour. On initial examination the cervix was 4 cm dilated and an ARM was performed which revealed meconium-stained liquor. Over the following 6 hours there were CTG abnormalities (variable decelebrations) but regular fetal blood sampling was normal (the pH was always > 7.25). The baby (male, weighing 3995 g) was delivered by ventouse with a cord pH of 7.23 and Apgars of 7 and 8.

Some 20 minutes after delivery the mother was holding the baby when she called for help and said that he had become limp. The paediatric SHO who had examined the baby at delivery came over, blew in the baby's face and receiving no response, did it again. The baby responded and the paediatric SHO told the mother that the baby was fine — she was just not used to newborn babies. Ten minutes later the senior midwife came into the room and found the baby to be dead. Resuscitation was attempted but failed.

A postmortem was subsequently discussed and agreed to, but there will be no results for several weeks. Initial examination of the baby in the ward was normal.

Role-player's instructions

You are very angry. You were happy with the obstetric management but you are not happy that your post-delivery concerns were not taken seriously. You are quite withdrawn and have been crying a lot since the baby died. You look and feel dreadful, and have had little sleep. You want to know:

1. ***Why did the baby die?***
2. ***Why was your concern not taken seriously?***
3. ***What did the postmortem show?***

You are considering suing the hospital.

Examiner's instructions

At this station you are examining the candidate's ability to counsel a woman after an unexpected neonatal death. The candidate also has to deal with the woman's anger and frustration about the tragic events surrounding the birth of her first child, her criticism of other doctors, and her intention to complain or possibly, sue. Marks should be allocated for the following features:

- Introduction: **5**
  - — Offer of sympathy
  - — Encourages mother to talk
  - — Eye contact
  - — Body language
  - — Use of appropriate language
- Sympathetic/caring approach: **5**
  - — Allows the patient to ask questions
  - — Sensitive to patient's distress
  - — Would they like to see baby again/photos?
  - — Book of remembrance
- Explains postmortem procedure in a non-medical way **2**
- Does not incriminate colleagues or assign blame **2**
- Arranging counselling **2**
- Asks about physical well-being **2**
- Funeral arrangements/birth registration **2**
- Home arrangements? **2**
- Offers future meeting. **2**

The following assessment and marking are done by the role-player:

- Caring/sympathetic approach **1**
- Trying to defuse situation **1**

• Understood the postmortem	**1**
• Would feel happy to return for further discussion	**2**
• Feels the candidate is being truthful/not hiding something.	**1**
Total mark out of 30: divide by 3 for final mark	

STATION 2.7

Labour ward management — preparatory station

Candidate's instructions

You are the registrar on call for the delivery unit. You have just arrived for the handover at 8.30 a.m. On the delivery unit board provided you will find brief summaries on the 10 women on the delivery suite.
The staff available today are:

- An obstetric SHO in her fourth month of GP training
- A third-year specialist anaesthetic registrar
- A consultant on call who is in his gynaecology clinic and who is not keen on being disturbed unless absolutely necessary
- Six midwives: SW is in charge. She and MC can suture episiotomies.

You have 15 minutes in which to decide what tasks need to be done, in which order they should be done, and who should be allocated to each task. At the next station you will discuss your decisions and your reasoning with an examiner. You will be awarded marks for your ability to manage the delivery suite.

DELIVERY UNIT BOARD

Room	Name	Para	Gestation	Liquor	Epidural	Syntocinon	Comments	Midwife
1	Neville	1+1	41			Yes	Normal delivery; hysterectomy for massive PPH; 1830 night before10 units transfused	SW
2	Barnes	2+0	T+9	Clear	No	No	7 cm at 0800; domino	Com/MW
3	Haig	0+0	39	Intact	No	No	Spont. labour; 4 cm at 0400; 5 cm at 0815	SW
4	Ferguson	0+0	28				Dr to see ? prem labour	MC
5	Milne	0+0	41	Mec	Yes	No	Fully dilated at 0630	VM
6	Shirodkar	1+0 (LSCS)	T+2	Clear	No	No	Trial of scar. ARM at 0300; FBS at 0600 — pH 7.29; 6 cm at 0600	DB
7	Murray	0+3	15				Routine admission for cervical suture	VM
8	Barton	0+0	39				Delivered; needs suturing	PL
9	Green	2+0	T+6	Intact	No	No	Spont. labour; 3 cm at 0650	MC
10	Armitage	0+0	26	Intact	No	No	In-utero transfer; IVF twins; PET	PL

STATION 2.8

Labour ward management — examination station

Marks

Examiner's instructions

The candidate has 15 minutes to explain the following:

1. The tasks which need to be done on the delivery suite.
2. The order in which the candidate decides they should be done and which staff should be allocated to each task.

1. **Tasks to be done:** **10**

- *Room 1* Review BP, urine output, pain relief, blood loss, general postop. Condition, drug regimen, IV fluids. Check Hb and clotting
- *Room 2* No action. Normal labour
- *Room 3* Needs assessment (1 cm increase in cervical dilatation in >4 hours). Doctor to examine. ? ARM, ? Syntocinon
- *Room 4* Needs assessment and more information. CTG
- *Room 5* Need to check progress and deliver
- *Room 6* Need to check CTG and progress. Confirm blood sent for FBC and group and save
- *Room 7* Check consent/fit for GA, needs FBC, group and save
- *Room 8* Needs suturing
- *Room 9* No action required
- *Room 10* Needs assessment of maternal and fetal well-being. Blood for U&E, urate, FBC, clotting, group and save. Decide if delivery required. Check neonatal cots and availability of senior anaesthetist.

2. **Priority of tasks and staff allocation:** **10**

- Urgent review by registrar in Rooms 6 and 5
- Semi-urgent review by registrar in Rooms 3 and 10
- SHO to assess patient in Room 4
- SHO and anaesthetist to see patient in Room 10 in first instance

- Routine review in Room 1 by SHO and anaesthetist
- Non-urgent review in Room 7
- Midwife to suture patient in Room 8
- No need for doctor in Rooms 2 and 9.

Total mark out of 20: divide by 2 for final mark

STATION 2.9

Mild endometriosis

Marks

Candidate's instructions

A 31-year-old patient with a 3-year history of primary infertility was fully investigated and only mild endometriosis was detected. Her partner had a normal seminal fluid analysis. *How would you proceed?*

Examiner's instructions

The marks should be awarded as follows:

- Mild endometriosis is associated with reduced fertility. This finding should not therefore be ignored and the case should not be treated as 'unexplained'. **1**
- Ablation of endometriotic lesions (diathermy/laser) is effective in increasing monthly pregnancy rate by up to 6% per cycle. **2**
- Danazol is not effective in increasing fertility either during or in the months after treatment. **1**
- Gonadotrophin-releasing hormone agonists are also ineffective. **1**
- There is a high chance of spontaneous pregnancy — up to 50% in the following 2 years (i.e. 2–3% per cycle). **2**
- Superovulation ± intrauterine insemination (IUI) will lead to a pregnancy rate of about 10% per cycle. **1**
- IVF will lead to a pregnancy rate of about 30% per cycle. **1**
- Presentation and examiner's discretion. **1**

Total mark out of 10

STATION 2.10

Hormone replacement therapy

	Marks

Candidate's instructions

A 48-year-old woman is to undergo total abdominal hysterectomy and bilateral salpingo-oophorectomy for heavy periods. What is your advice to her about hormone replacement therapy?

Examiner's instructions

The following points should be covered and marks allocated accordingly:

	Marks
• Vasomotor and other short-term symptoms	2
• Cardio-protective effect	2
• Osteoporosis	2
• The risk of thromboembolism is increased threefold, from 10 per 100 000 women per year to 30 per 100 000 women per year	2
• The risk of breast cancer is thought to be increased by a factor of 0.023 per year of use. The background incidence of breast cancer in women aged between 50 and 70 years is 45 cases per 1000. Use of HRT for 5 years is associated with an extra two cases of breast cancer being diagnosed by the age of 70. Use for 10 years is associated with an extra 6 cases, and for 20 years an extra 12 cases, per 1000 women	4
• Alternatives to oestrogen (e.g. SERMs)	2
• The fact that starting HRT is the patient's own decision, however useful the doctor thinks it is	4
• Presentation and examiner's discretion.	2

Total mark out of 20: divide by 2 for final mark

ORAL ASSESSMENT EXAMINATION

3

STATION 3.1

Progestogen-IUCD

Marks

Candidate's instructions

You will be provided with a Mirena coil and asked to identify it and discuss its therapeutic uses and possible unwanted effects.

Examiner's instructions

- A good candidate should identify the object as a progestogen-containing/releasing IUCD or as a Mirena or Progestasert (or other brand name) **2**
- If identified as IUCD only. **0**

If the candidate fails to identify the coil correctly, inform him that it is a progestogen-containing/releasing IUCD.

- A good candidate should know:
  - — Effective for 3–5 years **1**
  - — Contraceptive effectiveness similar to female sterilization (failure rate 2–3 per 1000; Pearl index 0.14). **1**
- Unwanted effects:
  - — Irregular menstrual and intermenstrual bleeding which subsides within 3–6 months **1**
  - — Follicular cysts/premenstrual symptoms in progestogen-sensitive women. **1**

Ask the candidate about the non-contraceptive uses of progestogen-releasing IUCDs:

- Management of menorrhagia — 86% reduction in blood loss after 3 months and 97% reduction after 12 months **1**
- Effective treatment for severe dysmenorrhoea **1**
- Effective treatment for uterine fibroids/endometriosis **1**
- Opposition to oestrogens or oestrogen-like substances, e.g. tamoxifen, HRT. **1**

Total mark out of 10

STATION 3.2

Day-case surgery — preparatory station

Candidate's instructions

You are working in a gynaecology unit which does not provide day-case surgery (DCS). You have been asked to give a talk to your clinical, nursing and managerial colleagues about the advantages and disadvantages of establishing such a service. You have 15 minutes to prepare this talk, and you will be asked to present it at the next station.

You have a maximum of three (A4 size) acetate sheets (these will be provided in the exam).

STATION 3.3

Day-case surgery — examination station

Marks

Examiner's instructions

The following points should be included, and marks allocated accordingly:

1. ***Advantages of DCS*:** 5

- Operations cost less than inpatient care. The day unit is closed at night and weekends thereby saving 'hotel' services and nurses' salaries.
- Elective admissions are not cancelled when emergency cases 'block' their beds.
- Day-surgery nurses are easier to recruit because of convenient working hours.
- Day surgery is less stressful and socially disruptive for patients.
- Hospital-acquired infections are less common.
- Inpatient surgical waiting lists can be reduced.

2. ***Disadvantages of DCS*:** 5

- Surgery may have to be postponed if medical or other problems are detected on the day of admission.
- Postoperative sequelae (e.g. pain) still occur and may persist after the patient has gone home.
- Postoperative overnight stay or readmission may be necessary because of unexpected complications.

3. ***Selection of patients*:** 5

- The patient should be fit and healthy, with no intercurrent medical disease which limits activity or is incapacitating (i.e. American Society of Anesthesiologists Classes 1 and 2).
- The patient must not be grossly obese.
- There must be no history of anaesthetic problems.
- There must be a suitable adult to accompany the patient home following surgery.
- The patient must have adequate support at home for 24 hours postoperatively.

- The patient's mental attitude towards illness and pain is important.
- The patient must be well informed, and surgical and nursing time has to be spent in the outpatient clinic informing the patient.

4. ***Selection of operation*:** 5

- Operations suitable for DCS are those which have low rates of postoperative complications and pain requiring more than simple oral analgesics (*The candidate is required to give examples and justify them*).

Total mark out of 20: divide by 2 for final mark

STATION 3.4

Counselling for hysterectomy — role-play

Candidate's instructions

Mrs Sloan is a 44-year-old woman who is having considerable problems with menorrhagia, which has failed to respond to medical treatment. She developed an iron-deficiency anaemia (haemoglobin 8.2 g/dl) which responded to oral iron. Over the last few years she has developed fairly severe secondary dysmenorrhoea which now does not respond to simple analgesics. Pelvic examination indicates a mobile tender uterus with no evidence of pelvic fibroids and no ovarian enlargement or tenderness. Transvaginal ultrasound examination showed no abnormality. She has always had normal cervical cytology.

You have offered her a hysterectomy and she wishes time to consider. She is anxious about the post-operative recovery. She mentions that a friend has told her that the operation ruins your sex life, gives you hot flushes and makes you incontinent.

How would you advise her?

Role-player's instructions

You are Mrs Sloan, a 44-year-old bank clerk, and you have been having increasing problems with heavy uncontrollable periods over the last 5 years. The menstrual loss has become so great that you have to take time away from work, and your periods are socially embarrassing. Recently your periods have been accompanied by severe menstrual cramps and you have been using painkillers to cope. You have been treated with several types of tablets in an attempt to control the menstrual loss, without much success. Other than your period problems you have no significant medical illnesses and are not on any treatment.

The doctor you are about to meet has offered you a hysterectomy and although you appreciate that this may solve your problems, you are concerned about how you might be after the operation. A friend of yours has had a difficult time since a hysterectomy and has been depressed. Your friend has told you that the operation ruins your sex life, gives you hot flushes and makes you incontinent. You would like some information and reassurance that this will not happen to you.

You are concerned and are looking for information that will help you make a decision. You appreciate that you cannot continue with the situation as it is at present.

Examiner's instructions

This is an interactive station which will assess the candidate's ability to counsel and give information to a patient who is trying to make a choice about whether she should undergo a total abdominal hysterectomy. The patient is an intelligent woman who simply requires clear, relevant information, given in a sympathetic manner, which would assist her in making her choice.

Marks should be allocated as indicated below:

- Approach to the patient and her partner **2**
- Shows understanding and sympathetic approach **2**
- Appropriate use of language (no medical jargon) **2**
- Good eye contact **2**
- Reviews the indications for hysterectomy: **3**
  - — Severe bleeding, resultant anaemia
  - — Secondary dysmenorrhoea
  - — Failure of conservative therapy
- Type of hysterectomy: abdominal/vaginal **2**
- Ablative techniques not suitable (because of dysmenorrhoea/ uterine pain) **2**
- Conservation of ovaries **2**
- The candidate should also discuss: **10**
  - — Postoperative discomfort
  - — Recovery — in hospital for approximately 5 days and then at home for up to 10–12 weeks
  - — Lifting — no heavy lifting for 3–6 weeks, increase gradually
  - — Exercise — after 4–6 weeks, also light housework
  - — Back to work — in 6–12 weeks
  - — Sex life, intercourse
  - — Urinary problems — postoperative urgency but this is usually temporary

— Menopause

— Premenstrual syndrome may continue

— Weight gain not directly related to operation

— No loss of femininity

• Role-player's assessment. 3

Total mark out of 30: divide by 3 for final mark

STATION 3.5	
Kielland's forceps	Marks

Candidate's instructions

You will be given an instrument (a pair of Kielland's forceps). You will be awarded marks for correct assembly of the instrument and for correct answers on its use.

Examiner's instructions

Mark the candidate on the assembly of the instrument and on his answers to questions on its use.

1. ***Assembly*:** **5**
   - Matches pair and assembles correctly
   - Correctly describes the special features of Kielland's forceps.
2. ***Precautions before application*:** **5**
   - Full dilatation
   - Cephalic, with position and presentation known
   - Fetal head in mid-cavity or below
   - Analgesia
   - Ruptured membranes
   - Empty bladder
   - Note: *the episiotomy is not done before application.*
3. ***Method of application*:** **5**
   - Correct procedure should be described.
4. ***Action the candidate would take if*:** **5**
   - Blades will not lock
   - Brisk blood loss after application
   - Fails to rotate with finger pressure only
   - Fails to descend on traction
   - Brisk PPH occurs.

Total mark out of 20: divide by 2 for final mark

STATION 3.6

Perineal tear

Marks

Candidate's instructions

A primiparous patient has just delivered a 3.89 kg baby spontaneously per vaginam. The third stage is complete without complication. The midwife who supervised the delivery believes there to be a third-degree tear and has asked for your help. Discuss your management.

Examiner's instructions

The candidate should:

1. Know how to define perineal tears.
2. Explain how to establish the diagnosis and display an understanding of the anatomy.
3. Know how to repair the damage.
4. Be able to prescribe correct aftercare.
5. Understand the functional implications of sphincter damage and dysfunction and explain to the patient what has happened and the implications for future deliveries.

These questions should be marked as follows:

1. ***What do you understand by a third-degree perineal tear?*** **3**
   - English definition: sphincter and anal mucosal damage
   - American definition: sphincter disruption
   - Fourth-degree: sphincter disruption plus mucosal damage.
2. ***How would you make the diagnosis?*** **2**
   - Inspection — defect in external sphincter
   - PR — loss of tone, retraction of sphincter (may not be clear with epidural).
3. ***How would you repair the tear?*** **10**
   - Involve consultant in theatre
   - Good lighting
   - Assistance
   - Good anaesthesia
   - Antibiotic cover (anaerobes)
   - PDS suture (not catgut)

- Overlap technique may be advantageous; end-to-end customary
- Careful check for sutures/damage in anal mucosa (fistula formation)
- Consider involving a colorectal surgeon.

4. ***What instructions would you give for post operative care?*** **5**
   - Laxative (lactulose)
   - Bulking agent
   - Antibiotics
   - General obs (temp.)
   - Postnatal follow-up.

5. ***What would you explain to the patient?*** **5**
   - Explanation of events
   - Frequency of this occurrence (sphincter damage more common than recognized — 20% in normal delivery and 80% in forceps delivery, in ultrasound studies)
   - Repair usually successful — incontinence uncommon
   - Urgency may be due to other effects of delivery, e.g. pudendal nerve damage
   - Vaginal delivery not contraindicated in future deliveries
   - Episiotomy may be advisable, although there is no hard evidence to show that this is protective
   - Caesarean delivery, with its morbidity, and mortality not warranted in light of current evidence on these grounds alone.

Total mark out of 25: divide by 2.5 for final mark and around down part of mark

STATION 3.7

Vaginal discharge

Marks

Candidate's instructions

You have received the following letter from a GP:

> Dear Colleague,
>
> Please would you see this 23-year-old student who is complaining of a persistent, offensive, green vaginal discharge. A cervical smear taken last year was reported as normal and a high vaginal swab taken recently by the practice nurse showed 'no significant growth'.
>
> Many thanks for you help . . .

Discuss with the examiner how you would proceed with the consultation and what tests you would like to perform.

Examiner's instructions

1. ***Relevant points the candidate should elicit from the examiner when discussing the history*:**

   - The patient is sexually active and uses Microgynon-30. **2**
   - She has regular periods, LMP was 3 weeks ago. **2**
   - She is in a stable relationship, but has had previous partners. **2**
   - She denies any history of pelvic infection, has never been pregnant and is otherwise fit and well. **2**
   - The discharge is worst during the first two weeks of her cycle and it does not itch. **2**
   - She believes that the smell is stronger following sexual intercourse. This is embarrassing her and making her reluctant to have intercourse. **2**

2. ***Examination and investigations*:**

- Examination of the external genitalia for signs of inflammation and/or excoriation. **2**
- Speculum examination, including visualization of the cervix which reveals an ectropion with a moderate, non-offensive discharge. **2**
- High vaginal swab (HVS) in universal medium for *T. vaginalis*, *Gardnerella, Bacteroides, Candida* etc. **4**
- Endocervical swab in universal medium for *N. gonorrhoeae*. **3**
- Endocervical swab in appropriate medium for chlamydia. **3**
- Bedside tests for bacterial vaginosis (BV):
  - — pH: HVS wiped onto narrow-range pH paper (pH > 5 suggestive of BV) **2**
  - — Amine test: HVS wiped onto slide and treated with KOH (fishy odour characteristic of BV) **1**
  - — Wet smear plus Gram's stain for cells characteristic of BV. **1**
- Repeat smear if considering cryocautery to cervix. **1**
- Bimanual examination to exclude obvious cervical excitation and hydrosalpinx. **1**

3. ***Treatment*:**

- If bedside tests suggest BV, treat with metronidazole (oral/p.v.) or clindamycin (p.v.). **2**
- Treat swab results as appropriate. **2**
- Refer to GUM clinic as appropriate. **2**
- If all swabs and smear normal, offer cervical cautery. **2**

Total mark out of 40: divide by 4 for final mark.

STATION 3.8

Breech presentation pamphlet — preparatory station

This is a preparatory station. You are asked to comment on the quality of the pamphlet supplied. It has been produced to inform patients who have a breech presentation about the condition and what options are open to them. Critically appraise the pamphlet and discuss it with the examiner in the next station. Indicate how you would improve it.

BREECH BABIES AND THEIR DELIVERY

Your baby is sitting bottom-first. Only about 3% of babies do this. It does not necessarily mean that there is an abnormality. Your doctors and midwives will be ready to answer any questions. This information sheet will give you some basics.

Why does it happen?

In most cases we never know. Sometimes the placenta lies in the lower part of the womb, preventing the baby's head from engaging. Rarely your pelvis may be inadequate to allow the head to engage, making it more likely that the bottom will come first.

What difference does it make?

Usually, the most difficult part of a baby to deliver is its head. It is also the part over which we take most care. When babies present head-first we get warning of mechanical problems and can take measures to get round them, e.g. caesarean section. With the bottom coming first, this may not be the case and once we have delivered the body, we are committed to complete vaginal delivery. Furthermore, once the umbilicus is delivered, the baby's oxygen supply is cut off until the baby can breathe spontaneously, i.e. after delivery of the head. Any delay can result in lack of oxygen. We therefore have to be confident that delivery is going to be straightforward if we go for a vaginal birth.

Is there anything that can be done to correct matters?

The baby can be turned in the womb. This is known as 'external cephalic version' (ECV). Usually, this is done on the Delivery Suite so that any complications can be handled, e.g. emergency caesarean section can be performed if the baby becomes distressed. If the ECV is successful, delivery is likely to take place as if the baby had *always* been headfirst. If it is not, then a decision will have to be made about caesarean section or vaginal delivery.

Vaginal birth* vs *caesarean section

At the present time there are no strong indicators for which is best. Vaginal birth carries uncertainties, particularly for the baby. We would normally advise continuous fetal heart rate monitoring and epidural analgesia throughout the labour. Caesarean section, on the other hand, is more risky for the mother. Ultimately, the choice is yours, and discussion about your particular circumstances with your midwife or obstetrician would be wise.

STATION 3.9

Breech presentation pamphlet — examination station

Marks

Examiner's instructions

The candidate should be aware of:

- Basic principles of effective written communication
- The document's good and bad points
- Factual inaccuracy or inadequacy.

The candidate should be awarded the following marks for his assessment of the pamphlet:

1. ***General points*:** 5

   - Short and to-the-point (perhaps too short)
   - Generally uses simple English but not always. Some use of technical jargon (placenta, engagement)
   - Is there bias? — tendency to use words with negative connotations (e.g. 'pelvis may be *inadequate*')
   - No date or name of person or organisation responsible for publication
   - Diagrams/pictures would aid clarity.

2. **Introductory, *Why does it happen?* and *What difference does it make?* paragraphs:** 5

   - Incidence correct for *term* — no mention of gestation
   - Does not go into possibilities such as uterine anomaly or fetal anomaly. This may have been deliberate but candidate should discuss
   - Does not mention investigations which could be done to give more information (ultrasound: placental site, check for fetal anomaly; check for extension of the neck, weight estimate (greater or less than 4 kg)) or tests which do *not* help (pelvimetry (erect lateral) of no value)
   - Tends to emphasize the *problems* without balancing this by information about what happens in most cases of properly managed breech delivery.

3. ***Is there anything that can be done to correct matters?* (ECV) paragraph:** **5**

- Rather negative
- Does not give full explanation (candidate should be able to do so)
- When? — 37 weeks (proposed trial for earlier version); done without anaesthesia; role of tocolytics (? of value in nulliparous patients)
- No indication given of likely success (60%)
- No indication given of complication rate (1%. No babies lost in published series — therefore safe)
- Recommended policy of professional bodies on basis of evidence; Halves the need for caesarean section.

4. ***Vaginal birth* vs *caesarean section*:** **5**

The pamphlet is out of date as it reflects the state of knowledge prior to the publication of the report of the Planned Caesarean Section Versus Planned Vaginal Birth for Term Breech, Multicentre Randomised Trial in October 2000. This trial showed that perinatal mortality, neonatal mortality or serious neonatal morbidity were significantly lower for planned caesarean section in comparison with planned vaginal delivery (relative risk 0.33). In addition, there were no differences between both groups in terms of maternal mortality or serious maternal morbidity.

Total mark out of 20: divide by 2 for final mark

STATION 3.10

Fluid therapy in PET

Marks

Candidate's instructions

Outline the principles of fluid therapy in severe pre-eclampsia.

Examiner's instructions

The following points should be discussed and marks awarded as follows:

- Intravascular volume is depleted compared with normal pregnancy. **1**
- Fluid shifts precipitate pulmonary oedema. **1**
- Oliguria occurs for a brief period following delivery and glomerular endotheliosis resolves spontaneously. **1**
- Need to monitor fluid administration by: **3**
  - — Meticulous attention to fluid balance and urine output
  - — Clinical state of patient
  - — Oxygen saturation
  - — Occasionally CVP (a reading of 5 mmHg in a woman with no known heart disease represents a full circulating compartment)
  - — Pulmonary artery catheterization.
- No advantage of colloid over crystalloid. **1**
- As pre-eclampsia is commonly accompanied by a capillary leak syndrome the effect of infused colloid or crystalloid tends to be transient as both fluids can escape into the extravascular space. **1**
- Rapid intravenous crystalloid administration may lower colloidal osmotic pressure (COP) by dilution of plasma proteins and thus increase the difference in COP between the intravascular and interstitial spaces. This promotes fluid shifts into the interstitial space and increases the risk of overt pulmonary oedema. **1**
- More mothers die from the adult respiratory distress syndrome (ARDS) that complicates over-transfusion, fluid load and pulmonary oedema than from renal failure due to hypovolaemia. **1**

Total mark out of 10

ORAL ASSESSMENT EXAMINATION

4

STATION 4.1

Poor obstetric history — role-play

Candidate's instructions

You have received the following letter from a GP:

> Dear Colleague,
>
> Please would you see this 35–year-old teacher for booking. Her LMP was 12/01/1999. Of note, she had a miscarriage at 20 weeks in 1991 followed by a successful pregnancy in 1992. This was complicated by a DVT at around 32 weeks gestation.
>
> I would be happy to share care in the usual way,
>
> Yours sincerely . . .
>
> *Enclosed*:
>
> Report of pelvic ultrasound on 22/06/00 for – Selima Ali (d.o.b. 22/07/65)
>
> There is a singleton intrauterine pregnancy
> CRL = 45 mm = 12 weeks 1 day
> Fetal heart activity seen

Take a history from this patient, counsel her regarding appropriate investigations and plan her further antenatal care.

Role-player's instructions

This was a planned pregnancy. Your partner is the father of your previous children and you and your partner are not blood relations. You had been using barrier contraception. You have been taking folic acid, but no other medication and are fit and well.

You do not remember much about the pregnancy loss in 1991: you had had some bleeding in the early part of the pregnancy and remember presenting with bleeding and pain at around five months. You had a normal delivery but the baby 'was too small' to live. No one told you a reason for the loss.

You also recall some bleeding during the subsequent pregnancy in 1992. At about 32 weeks into the second pregnancy you needed hospital treatment, with a drip and injections, for a clot in your left leg. You were induced at term because the doctors were worried about the baby being small, and had a vaginal delivery of a healthy boy weighing 5 lb 11 oz. He is alive and well. You needed to take warfarin tablets after the delivery for several months.

These pregnancies took place at another hospital.

You have no other medical or family history of note.

Examiner's instructions

The following points should be noted and discussed, and marks awarded as follows:

1. ***Communication***:

- Introduction 2
- Eye contact 2
- Making the patient feel at ease 2
- Allowing the patient to ask questions. 2

2. ***History-taking***:

- Pregnancy loss, including history of bleeding 2
- Second pregnancy, including bleeding, DVT, induction, small baby 2
- Family history — no other clotting problems? 2

3. ***Counselling***:

- Routine tests including FBC, electrophoresis, blood group and antibodies, syphilis, hepatitis and HIV 2
- Investigation of possible thrombophilia 2
- Downs syndrome screening 2
- Offer of detailed (anomaly) scan. 2

4. ***Pregnancy plan***:

- Write to hospitals for information about previous pregnancies 2
- Liaise with haematologist regarding DVT prophylaxis 2
- Review with results (after about 2 weeks — may need aspirin/heparin if thrombophilia detected) 2
- Serial scans in view of pregnancy loss and IUGR. 2

Total mark out of 30: divide by 3 for final mark

STATION 4.2

Critical incident monitoring — preparatory station

Candidate's instructions

Monitoring the frequency of critical clinical incidents (or adverse events) is an important part of ensuring a high quality of obstetric clinical practice. Your unit wishes to introduce a scheme which automatically reports critical and or adverse incidents associated with labour and its outcome.

Discuss with the examiner at the next station how you would develop and use a list of critical incidents or markers to monitor intrapartum care in your maternity unit.

STATION 4.3

Critical incident monitoring — examination station

Marks

Examiner's instructions

The following points should be discussed, and the marks awarded as indicated:

1. The candidate should ***understand the concept*** of critical or adverse clinical incidents. In order to improve clinical standards and to monitor clinical practice, many maternity units are devising a list of adverse clinical incidents and are monitoring the frequency at which such events are occurring. If an unusual pattern or increased frequency of events is detected, an investigation could be initiated. Single life-threatening events such as eclampsia or severe antepartum or postpartum haemorrhage would also initiate a clinical review. **2**

2. The candidate should have a ***logical approach*** to the problem and use a logical classification of factors such as the following types of categories: **4**

   - Labour
   - Induction of labour
   - First stage
   - Second stage
   - Third stage
   - Puerperium
   - Maternal outcome
   - Fetal outcomes
   - Staffing
   - Anaesthetic.

3. ***Examples of main critical or adverse incidents.*** (This is not an exclusive list: others may be included.)

a) Labour: **10**

- Failed induction of labour
- Use of prostaglandin agents in a second 24 hours
- Induction delivery interval > 24 hours

- Syntocinon infusion > 100 iu/24 hours
- Uterine hypertonus — initiation of treatment
- Precipitate labour (3 cm to full dilation < 2 hours)
- Malpresentation in labour
- Prolapsed cord in labour
- Fetal distress (non-reassuring CTG).

b) Method of Delivery: **10**

- Decision to caesarean section intervals
  < 30, 30–45, 45+ minutes
- Ruptured uterus
- Failed forceps
- Failed vacuum extraction
- Vacuum extraction duration > 15 minutes.

c) Postpartum: **10**

- Third/fourth-degree tear
- Intrapartum blood transfusion
- Haemorrhage (antepartum or postpartum)
- Retained placenta, retained placental tissue
- Hb < 8.0 g or fall of 3 g
- Wound breakdown — perineal or caesarean section
- Return to theatre
- Maternal admission to ICU
- Unexpected maternal pyrexia
- Trauma to other internal organs.

d) Fetal outcomes: **10**

- Apgar score < 5 at 1 minute ; < 5 at 5 minutes
- Unexpected admission to SCBU
- Cord blood pH < 7.1
- Undiagnosed fetal anomaly

- Perinatal sepsis
- Fetal trauma or incision.

e) Anaesthetic/pain relief: **10**

- Epidural difficulties
- Failure to receive (staffing problems)
- Dural tap
- Dural headache
- Conversion to GA
- Failed intubation.

f) Staffing problems: **4**

- Failure to respond to bleep/unable to contact
- Staff fully committed and so unavailable to respond (e.g. in theatre)
- Insufficient staff (less than complement).

Total mark out of 60: divide by 6 for final mark

STATION 4.4

Menorrhagia on tamoxifen — Role-play

Candidate's instructions

You have received the following letter from a GP:

Dear Colleague,

Please would you see this 47-year-old lawyer who is suffering from menorrhagia. On examination I felt the uterus was enlarged and an ultrasound scan has confirmed a fibroid uterus (report enclosed).

Mrs Smith had a mastectomy 2 years ago for cancer of the breast and is currently taking tamoxifen.

Yours sincerely . . .

Enclosed: Report on pelvic ultrasound on 22/06/00 for Angela Smith (d.o.b. 12/04/53)

Anteverted uterus, which is bulky in appearance, measuring 20 x 15 x 10 cm. There are several areas that are suggestive of fibroids, the largest of which is situated at the fundus and measures 12x8x8 cm. Unable to visualize the endometrium due to multiple fibroids. Both ovaries were seen and appeared normal (left measuring 33 x 20 x 13 mm, right measuring 29 x 19 x 14 mm). No adnexal masses or free fluid seen.

Take a history from this patient. The examiner will advise you of the findings of any examination you would like to perform. You must then counsel the patient regarding the differential diagnosis, options for further investigation, and treatment.

Examiner's instructions

The following points should be assessed, and marks awarded as follows:

1. ***Communication***

- Introduction **1**
- Eye contact **1**
- Making the patient feel at ease **1**
- Allowing the patient to ask questions. **1**

2. ***History-taking***

- Open questions **1**
- Menstrual history (including smear history). **4**

(The Role-player will give the following information:LMP, regular cycle, no IMB or PMB, flooding, affecting work, severe cramps).

- Obstetric history (especially female children) **1**
- PMH (breast cancer, follow-up, expected duration of tamoxifen therapy) **1**
- Drug history (contraception, previous treatment for menorrhagia, allergies) **1**
- Family history (particularly other female relatives and breast, endometrium, ovary and colon cancers). **1**

3. ***Examination***

- General condition (fitness for surgery) **1**
- Abdominal and bimanual (mobility of uterus, presence of nodules suggestive of Ca) **2**
- Speculum (look for polyps/cervical lesion) and outpatient endometrial biopsy, e.g. Pipelle's (plus smear if not up-to-date) **2**
- FBC (if not had one recently). **1**

4. ***Management***

- If Pipelle normal:
  - — Haematinics if anaemic 2
  - — Do nothing and keep under review, however problems likely to persist and may get worse 1
  - — Medical treatment (tranexamic acid) and keep under review 1
  - — Explain that treatments such as Mirena and endometrial ablation are unlikely to be effective given the size of the uterus 1
  - — Offer TAH and BSO 1
- Pipelle equivocal:
  - — Will need hysteroscopy and curettage or TAH + BSO 2
- Pipelle abnormal:
  - — Refer to gynae-oncologists. 4

5. ***Discussion of management with patient***

- Candidate should advise TAH + BSO on grounds of:
  - — Fibroids likely to grow, causing further problems with bleeding and making surgery more difficult 2
  - — Risk of malignant change within the fibroids (less than 0.5%) 1
  - — Ongoing risk of endometrial carcinoma from tamoxifen therapy, requiring ongoing follow-up and probably further investigations 1
  - — BSO advised on grounds of age (close to menopause, future risk of Ca ovary approx 1%) and history of Ca breast 2
- Candidate should discuss HRT (need to liaise with breast surgeons: preparations such as Raloxifene and Tibolone will not stimulate breast tissue but Raloxifene will not stop hot flushes) 1
- Candidate should advise removal of cervix where possible, given risk of continued problems with bleeding/endometrial stimulation by tamoxifen 1

- In view of early age of diagnosis of Ca breast, candidate should enquire about family history of other cancers as above, and discuss possible genetics referral for other female relatives (e.g. daughters, sisters). 1

Total mark out of 40: divide by 4 for final mark

STATION 4.5

Fetal anomaly counselling — role-play

Candidate's instructions

Mrs Patricia O'Reilly, a 30-year-old woman, presents in her first pregnancy. She has 15 weeks amenorrhoea, her menstrual cycle was regular and she was not using hormonal preparations prior to conception. An early ultrasound scan had confirmed a single fetus of a size corresponding to the period of gestation, 15 weeks.

Her sister (age 38, para 5) has just given birth to an infant with Down's syndrome and severe cardiac anomalies. She is very concerned about the risk of the fetus being abnormal.
How would you advise her?

Role-player's instructions

You are Mrs Patricia O'Reilly, a 30-year-old woman in your first pregnancy. You have a regular menstrual cycle and you are now 15 weeks pregnant. This was confirmed by an early scan. You have not been using the 'pill' or any other hormones.

Your sister, who is aged 38, has just given birth to a baby with Down's syndrome. The baby also has severe heart problems and is not expected to live. Her other children are normal.

You are very worried that your baby may be affected. You would like to know if there are any tests which can reassure you.

If necessary, you should ask about the scan and the 'amnio' test.

Examiner's instructions

This station aims to assess the candidate's ability to counsel effectively a patient who is concerned about a fetal anomaly. It is important that Mrs O'Reilly is made aware of and helped to understand the concept of "risk". She should be helped to understand the reliability and the limitations of intrauterine diagnosis and be given appropriate information to allow her to arrive at a decision as to whether to progress with fetal anomaly investigations. The consequences of the results, including termination of pregnancy, should be explained to her. The following points should be assessed, and marks awarded as follows:

- Empathetic approach: aware of patient's concerns and sensitivities **1**
- Use of non-technical language (absence of jargon) **1**
- Explanation of the procedures and risks involved **1**
- Explanation of the accuracy and reliability of the results and how they influence the patient's risk of abnormality **1**
- Assesses the basis of the patient's risk of the fetal anomaly of Down's syndrome: **1**

  — 1st degree relative with age-related Down's syndrome

  — Maternal age 30, no other risk of Down's syndrome

  — Explains that patient is at low risk, approximately 1 in 1000
- Explains use of ultrasound 'soft markers', e.g. nuchal translucency: **1**

  — NT < 3 mm: risk = 3x risk based on age alone

  — NT > 4 mm: risk = 18x risk based on age alone

  — NT > 6 mm: risk = 36x risk based on age alone

  — Explains that NT can adjust the risk but is *not* diagnostic
- Explains 'triple test' — venous blood sample measuring the three substances, AFP, E3 and β-hCG: can adjust the risk but is *not* diagnostic **1**
- Amniocentesis/cordocentesis with chromosomal analysis: diagnostic and gives a reliable result **1**
- Amniocentesis carries risk of fetal loss, approximately 1 in 300, and so would not be justified with the current level of risk **1**
- Explains that such invasive investigations may produce information which will require further action. Assesses whether the patient would be prepared to have a termination of pregnancy. If not, then should counsel against invasive investigations. **1**

Total mark out of 10

STATION 4.6

Borderline ovarian tumour — role-play

Candidate's instructions

An extra patient has been slotted in at the end of your clinic. She is a 34-year-old woman who underwent an emergency laparotomy and left oophorectomy two weeks ago for torsion of an ovarian cyst that was thought to be a dermoid. The histology has been reported as showing a borderline mucinous cystadenoma. The preoperative ultrasound had also suggested a 15 mm simple cyst on the *right* ovary that was not mentioned in the operation notes.

Take a history from this patient. The examiner will advise you of the findings of any examination you would like to perform. You must then counsel the patient regarding the differential diagnosis, options for further investigation, and treatment. You are given this sheet of patient notes:

Patient Notes: Mrs Mary Johnson (d.o.b. 13/4/66)

Past obstetric history

Two children: boy (age 9) and a girl (age 2). Both were normal vaginal deliveries. Family now complete.

Past gynaecological history

A four-year history of infertility prior to the birth of youngest child. A total of around 2 years treatment with clomifene. Now using condoms for contraception. Periods irregular, loss not heavy. Smear 3 years ago normal.

Past medical history

Mild asthma.

Drug history

Inhalers. No allergies.

Family history

Father alive and well.

Mother died of ovarian cancer age 64.

One sister age 31, who is alive and well.

Social history

Smokes 10/day.

Teacher.

Examiner's instructions

The following should be assessed, and marks awarded as follows:

1. ***Communication***:

- Introduction **1**
- Eye contact **1**
- Making the patient feel at ease **1**
- Allowing the patient to ask questions. **1**

2. ***History-taking***:

- Open questions **1**
- Obstetric history (especially female children, completed family) **1**
- Gynae history (especially infertility and clomifene use) **1**
- Family history (especially mother and sister). **1**

3. ***Examination***:

- Examine wound, check for lymphadenopathy. **1**

4. ***Counselling***:

- Nature of cyst — borderline malignancy **1**

2 Implication — uncertain malignant potential **1**

- Two management options:
  - — Pelvic clearance and HRT **1**
  - — Monitor with annual TV U/S and CA125 **1**
- Advantage of pelvic clearance is that it minimises risk of recurrence **1**
- Disadvantage of pelvic clearance is need for further surgery and for HRT **1**
- Disadvantage of conservative management is that there is no guarantee that a recurrent cancer will be picked up in time to allow curative surgery (screening is not yet evidence-based — merely the 'best we have') **2**

- In view of histology, family history, completed family and unknown efficacy of screening, pelvic clearance should be preferred option 1
- Advise that other female members of the family may be eligible for screening. 1

Total mark out of 20: divide by 2 for final mark

STATION 4.7

Down's syndrome baby

Marks

Candidate's instructions

You perform a lift-out delivery of a full-term baby after a prolonged second stage of labour. The labour has been otherwise uneventful. The baby pinks up and cries immediately. As you clamp the cord and observe the baby you recognize typical features of Down's syndrome. The mother is age 21 and had a low risk of Down's syndrome on screening. Discuss with the examiner what you would do and why.

Examiner's instructions

The following points should be discussed and marks awarded as indicated:

- The baby is pink, crying and well, so there is no need for immediate intervention. **2**
- Research has shown that parents' preference for being told news is that it should be done:
  - — To both parents together **1**
  - — In quiet and privacy **1**
  - — By the most senior clinical person available, usually a middle-grade or consultant paediatrician. **1**
- If the parent or parents express no specific immediate worry about the baby's normality, you should proceed with normal postpartum care (management of the third stage, stitches) and then inform your paediatric colleagues of your suspected diagnosis. They will review the baby clinically, interview parents within a few hours and send diagnostic chromosome samples. **2**
- Record your suspicions, and what you have done, in the case records. **1**
- Discuss your suspicions with the midwife caring for the mother and child. **1**
- If a parent shows immediate anxiety about the baby's normality you should express your shared concern and arrange for an early paediatric review. **1**

Total mark out of 10

STATION 4.8

Anaesthesia for vaginal hysterectomy

Marks

Candidate's instructions

A fit 50-year-old woman is to undergo a vaginal hysterectomy with anterior and posterior colporrhaphy. Discuss the anaesthetic options available to her.

Examiner's instructions

The following points should be discussed and awarded marks as indicated:

- Conventional general anaesthesia utilizing specific drugs for induction and maintenance of anaesthesia, muscle relaxation and analgesia. **2**
- Total intravenous anaesthesia utilizing the *same* drug for induction and maintenance of anaesthesia, adding a muscle relaxant and analgesics as required, but avoiding inhalation anaesthesia. **2**
- Regional techniques, either an epidural, a spinal or a combined spinal and epidural (CSE technique). If an epidural or CSE is inserted then the epidural component can be utilized for postoperative analgesia. **2**
- Any combination of the above, using regional anaesthesia as the analgesic component of a general anaesthetic. **2**
- Postoperative analgesia should also be discussed. Opiates will be required either in the form of intermittent injections, as an opiate infusion, or as PCA. Opiates could also be given intrathecally or epidurally if a regional technique is used. **2**

Total mark out of 10

STATION 4.9

Hepatitis B in pregnancy

Marks

Candidate's instructions

A 21-year-old woman who is 20 weeks pregnant is seen in the antenatal clinic. The results of her booking hepatitis screen are:

Hepatitis B surface antigen	positive
Hepatitis Be antigen	positive
Hepatitis B surface antibody	negative
Hepatitis Bc antibody	positive

Discuss your management with the examiner.

Examiner's instructions

The following points should be discussed and marks awarded as shown:

- This patient is highly infectious; the positive HBe AG indicating continuous viral replication. 1
- Modes of transmission are: blood-borne (transfusion), sexual intercourse, and splashing of blood or body fluids (e.g. amniotic fluid) onto open wounds or mucous membranes. 2
- With the patient's consent, the partner should be informed and offered screening. If he is negative, he should be immunized. Protected intercourse (condoms) should be used until immunity documented. 1
- The maximum risk of infection to the baby is at delivery due to swallowing of maternal blood/ amniotic fluid while passing through the birth canal. 1
- *Infected* babies will have a 90% chance of being chronic carriers. 1
- The risk of infection to the baby is significantly reduced with immunization, which should be both passive and active. Passive immunization is by immunoglobulins (within 12–24 hours of birth); active immunization is by HepB vaccine at birth (within 24 hours), and at 1 and 6 months. 1

- Breastfeeding is not contraindicated if the baby has been properly immunized. **1**
- The inside of the notes should be clearly labelled. The patient, together with all body substances such as blood samples and waste, should be treated as an infectious hazard. **1**
- Staff attending delivery should be properly equipped, i.e. water proof disposable gowns and masks, eye protection, double gloving for suturing, etc. **1**

Total mark out of 10

STATION 4.10

Sterilization in the luteal phase

Marks

Candidate's Instructions

You are the consultant doing the pre-operative ward round. A 35-year old woman, with three living children and a stable relationship is on the list for laparoscopic sterilization using Filshie clips. She has been seen previously in the clinic and properly counselled about the procedure and she has signed the appropriate consent form. She is fit and healthy, has had no previous operations, and her BMI is 22.

Explain to the examiner what you would discuss with the patient preoperatively.

Examiner's Instructions

The main aim of this station is to test the candidate's ability to manage a case of a patient presenting for sterilisation in the luteal phase, having had unprotected sexual intercourse in mid-cycle. The following points should be discussed, and the marks awarded as indicated :

- Enquiry about LMP, regularity of the cycle and current method of contraception. 3

The Examiner should prompt the candidate to ask about these if not done unprompted. Deduct 1 mark if prompted. The candidate is told that the cycle is usually 4/28, LMP was 16 days previously, and no contraception is being used.

- Enquiry about the last episode of unprotected sexual intercourse. 2

Again here the Examiner should prompt the candidate to ask about these if not done unprompted. Deduct 1 mark if prompted. The candidate is told that this was 4 days previously.

- Discussion about the risk of luteal-phase pregnancy in that situation, and the fact that applying a clip on the tube may actually precipitate an ectopic pregnancy (if the fertilized egg is still lateral to the clip in the tube). Explore the candidate's knowledge about luteal phase-pregnancy (accounts for about 30% of overall sterilisation failures) and the fact that 5% of women presenting for sterilization have been found to be pregnant in some studies. 4

The question states 'properly counselled'. The candidate should be told that the counselling included advice (and documentation) that a proper contraceptive should be used until the sterilisation had been performed.

- Performing a D&C at the same time does *not* guarantee that an intrauterine pregnancy will not occur. 2

- The patient is too late for hormonal postcoital contraception, and an IUCD, (although this can still be fitted) does not guarantee 100% against pregnancy. The risk of precipitating an ectopic pregnancy, mentioned earlier, still exists with postcoital contraception. 2

- Management options are: either to cancel the operation and reschedule during the follicular phase (or at any time in the cycle with reliable contraception), or to go ahead with the patient's full understanding that she may end up with an ectopic or an intrauterine pregnancy. Decision to reschedule should be courteously explained to the patient and documented in the notes. 5

The option of going ahead after informing the patient has been found indefensible medico-legally (as evidenced by a 1997 court case) and does not conform to good clinical practice. The examiner should ask directly what the candidate would do in such a situation, together with justification of the proposed action.

You have decided to reschedule the operation. The patient is unhappy and threatens to complain. What will you do?

- No change in decision. Proper documentation in the notes and perhaps filling in an incident form. 2

Total mark out of 20: divide by 2 for final mark

ORAL ASSESSMENT EXAMINATION

5

STATION 5.1

ASA classification

Marks

Candidate's instructions

Discuss with the examiner how you would classify the physical status of a patient who is going to have an operation that is suitable for day-case surgery.

Examiner's instructions

The following points should be discussed, and marks awarded as shown:

- Need for classification: physical evaluation of patients for suitability for day-case surgery involves the assignment of a physical-status category, based on history and examination. This acts as a useful 'language' for communication with colleagues. **5**
- The system in common use is that devised by the American Society of Anesthesiologists (ASA), in which patients are divided into five categories: **15**

  ASA 1 Normal healthy patient with no known organic, biochemical or psychiatric disease

  ASA 2 Patient with mild to moderate systemic disease

  ASA 3 Patient with severe systemic disease that limits normal activity

  ASA 4 Patient with severe systemic disease that is a consistent threat to life

  ASA 5 Patient who is moribund and unlikely to survive 24 hours.

- The estimated postoperative mortality rates for these categories are 0.06%, 0.4%, 4.3%, 23.4% and 50% respectively. **2**
- A drawback of this system is that it does not take the nature of the intended surgery into consideration. **2**
- Patients in categories ASA 1 and 2 are potentially suitable for day-case surgery.

The examiner should ask the candidate what other factors should be taken into consideration in addition to the nature of the operation and the physical status of the patient.

- Other factors in suitability for day-case surgery: **6**
  - — The patient must not be grossly obese
  - — There must be no history of anaesthetic problems
  - — There must be a suitable adult to accompany the patient home following surgery.
  - — The patient must have adequate support at home for 24 hours postoperatively
  - — The patient's mental attitude towards illness and pain is important
  - — The patient must be well informed, and surgical and nursing time has to be invested in the outpatient clinic informing the patient about the process.

Total mark out of 30: divide by 3 for final mark

STATION 5.2

Retained swab — role-play

Candidate's instructions

You are a consultant, seeing a 32-year-old barrister who is 6 weeks postnatal. You received a phone call from the A&E consultant yesterday informing you that this patient had attended with an offensive PV discharge and the SHO had removed a surgical swab from her vagina. As a result of this call you contacted the patient and asked her to attend today to discuss matters.

You have her hospital notes, which indicate that this was her first pregnancy. The antenatal course was unremarkable and you only saw her once at her booking visit: you were away at the time she delivered. She had gone into labour spontaneously at term. She had progressed spontaneously to 7 cm, when there appeared to have been some delay, with no progress over the following 3 hours. An ARM was performed and an epidural sited as she was becoming distressed. Syntocinon was begun 1 hour later as there had been no further progress. Two hours after the Syntocinon was started she was found to be fully dilated but the head was only at the level of the ischial spines. The

Patient Notes

02.15: ATSP. Pushing 1 hour, head not visible

CTG: FH 160, dips

O/E Ceph, +1 to spines, deflexed LOA, caput +, moulding +

For ventouse delivery

Operation notes:

— Lithotomy
— Swab, drape, catheter
— Brown silc-cup applied, pressure to 0.8
— Position checked — no skin trapped
— Good descent with traction, right medio-lateral episiotomy
— Head delivered with third contraction
— Baby girl (3.6 kg, Apgar 7 and 9) delivered with next contraction — cried — handed to paed.
— Placenta — CCT
— Epis. sutured in layers with vicryl
— EBL 1000 ml from episiotomy (uterus well contracted)
— Swabs and instruments correct
— For 2-unit Tx as pre-delivery Hb 9.5.

epidural was topped up and an hour allowed for descent, after which time she started pushing, with the head now felt to be below spines. An hour later delivery was not felt to be imminent and the fetal heart rate had risen from 140 to 160, with variable decelerations.

The registrar was called to review. From the notes she appears to have been a locum no longer employed by the Trust. She attended promptly and examined the patient. Her notes read as shown in the box on page 86.

She was transfused with two units of blood and discharged from hospital 2 days later with apparently normal lochia and a Hb of 110 g/L. It appears that a vaginal swab was taken on the day of discharge, which showed a heavy growth of *Bacteroides*. The GP was duly notified.

You must now counsel this patient.

Role-player's instructions

You are a barrister, appearing calm, but very angry. You have suffered with a continuous heavy, offensive vaginal discharge since you left hospital. You did in fact mention it to the midwife who discharged you. She took a swab but reassured you that it was normal.

The GP and midwife did visit in the first few days following discharge from hospital but they also reassured you that the loss was normal. You attended the surgery complaining of the discharge the following week. The GP did not examine you, but gave you some antibiotics. This did improve things, but the discharge came back within days of finishing the course. A student health visitor had also visited you and taken a swab, leading to the prescription of more antibiotics from the GP: This helped, once again, but the discharge rapidly returned. Eventually, in desperation, you had attended A & E. The attending doctor inserted a speculum and found a surgical swab, which he removed with great glee. He gave you yet another course of antibiotics.

You are going to sue for compensation. You have suffered needlessly with an embarrassing, horribly smelly discharge for six weeks; you have been fobbed off by midwives and your GP, none of whom had bothered to pass a speculum; and you are also concerned about your future fertility.

Examiner's instructions

The following should be assessed, and marked as follows:

1. ***Manner*:**
   - Introduction 1
   - Eye contact 1
   - Allowing patient to speak without undue interruption 1
   - Ability to avoid/diffuse confrontation. 2
2. ***Content*:**
   - Apology and explanation for not having seen patient during confinement 1
   - Sincere and unreserved apology regarding statement of fact (notification about the retained swab) 2
   - Enquiry as to the health of the patient 1
   - Ability to elucidate history from the patient 1
   - Explanation of events leading to retained swab — major haemorrhage, need for registrar to staunch bleeding with swabs etc. 2
   - Explanation that the person suturing is supposed to check all the swabs at the end of the procedure, and that the doctor had signed to say that they were correct 1
   - Acceptance that despite this, there is no other apparent reason for the swab to have been there and therefore that retention of the swab was negligent 1
   - Explanation to the patient that a full internal investigation will be performed and statements taken from those involved. Offer to discuss findings and action at a future date 2
   - Explanation of grievance procedure (write to the Chief Executive with complaint) 1
   - Reassurance about future fertility: offer follow-up with repeat swabs after present course of antibiotics. Offer HSG if there is delay in conception in the future 2
   - Ability to avoid passing precipitate judgment on other professionals before the full facts are made available. 1

Total mark out of 20: divide by 2 for final mark

STATION 5.3	
Familial ovarian cancer — role-play	Marks

Candidate's instructions

Mrs Jones is a 52-year-old woman who presents with anxiety about developing ovarian cancer. A friend of hers has recently died with the disease — she had had no symptoms prior to diagnosis, at which point the disease was already advanced. Mrs Jones wonders whether or not there are any tests that can be performed which might detect ovarian cancer or a risk of developing ovarian cancer. *How would you establish whether there is any increased risk in her case and advise her about screening tests and prophylaxis?*

Role-player's instructions

You are a 52-year-old woman who works in the School Meals Service. You were married at age 17 and have three grown-up children, two daughters and a son. You have a sister who emigrated to Australia 30 years ago, with whom you have had very little contact, but you do know that she had treatment for breast cancer last year. Your mother went to Australia 10 years ago to be near your sister: she died from cancer and although you are not sure, you believe it may have been cancer of the ovary.

You have been very well, you have had no operations and are not on any treatment.

A friend of yours has recently died from ovarian cancer. She had no symptoms prior to the diagnosis being made, at which point the disease was far advanced. Not only are you concerned about *her* death, but also about the fact that there appears to have been some deaths from cancer in your own family.

Examiner's instructions

This station aims to assess the candidate's knowledge of screening for ovarian cancer, its effectiveness and the implications for the patient and her family. The following should be discussed and marked as indicated:

- Should enquire about *family history and relevant personal history*
  - — History of ovarian, breast or bowel cancer in mother, aunts, sisters (i.e. first-degree relatives) 2
  - — Use of O/C pill and number of pregnancies. 2

- *Counselling* points should include:
  - — General lifetime risk of developing ovarian cancer is 1% **1**
  - — Most cases are sporadic **1**
  - — Increased risk if there is a family history. For example, there is a 3% lifetime risk if the patient is aged 52 with a mother having ovarian cancer at 65; increasing to 30% if two first-degree relatives have ovarian cancer. Risk is doubled if the patient has had breast cancer **2**
  - — Decreased risk with increasing number of pregnancies and previous contraceptive pill use **2**
  - — No current specific screening tests are available: both CA125 and transvaginal ultrasound are poorly predictive, but may be useful together **1**
  - — Genetic tests are available, e.g. presence of the BRCA1 gene. **1**
- Candidate should be aware that presymptomatic testing is available for cancer predisposition if there is a family history. However, he should make the patient aware of the practical and ethical problems: difficulties in obtaining life insurance, lack of proven benefit from intervention; and implications for offspring if she is a carrier. **2**

Counselling in Mrs Jones' case will depend on the type of cancer which her mother and sister had — what do you estimate Mrs Jones' risk to be?

- Risk approximately 30% **2**
- If increased risk based on history as above, the candidate should suggest:
  - — Follow-up at a screening clinic — using transvaginal ultra sound, CA125, BRCA1 **2**
  - — If the patient is high risk (> 30% or a BRCA1 gene carrier) consider oophorectomy, although this does not *eliminate* risk **2**

Total mark out of 20: divide by 2 for final mark

STATION 5.4	
Aortic stenosis in pregnancy	Marks

Candidate's instructions

A 20-year-old primigravida known to have aortic stenosis is booked for an elective caesarean section. Describe the underlying pathology, the rationale behind the choice of anaesthetic technique to be employed and which techniques can be offered.

Examiner's instructions

The following points should be discussed, and marks awarded as shown:

- This is likely to be a congenital aortic stenosis. Aortic stenosis is accompanied by left ventricular hypertrophy, myocardial ischaemia and a fixed cardiac output. **5**
- The rationale for using a particular anaesthetic technique is the maintenance of haemodynamic stability. *Acute after-load reduction* due to vasodilatation gives rise to decreased coronary perfusion and myocardial ischaemia as the hypertrophied myocardium is vulnerable to ischaemia. Tachycardia decreases ventricular filling time and hence decreases cardiac output. Hypovolaemia, bradycardia, peripheral vasodilatation, drugs causing myocardial depression and any other arrhythmias can lead to a decrease in cardiac output and cardiovascular collapse. *Fluid overload* can cause cardiac decompensation and pulmonary oedema. **10**
- Management: **5**
  - — Establish invasive monitoring — arterial line and CVP
  - — Ensure: no adverse heart rates, no hypotension, no hypertension, no fluid overloading
  - — Prophylaxis against bacterial endocarditis
  - — Nurse in a high-dependency area postoperatively.
- If haemodynamic stability is maintained, slow incremental epidural or subarachnoid anaesthesia, or cardiovascularly tailored general anaesthesia can be successfully administered. Avoided the single-shot spinal anaesthetic with its rapid sympathetic blockade, vasodilatation and decreased cardiac output. **5**

Total mark out of 25: divide by 2.5 for final mark and round down part of mark

STATION 5.5

Delivery suite priorities

Marks

Candidate's instructions

You are the registrar on call for the delivery suite. You have only one operating theatre available to you. There is one on-call anaesthetic registrar who is covered by his consultant.

You have been called to perform a manual removal of placenta on primiparous patient who has just delivered normally. As you are preparing to see this patient your experienced SHO informs you that a second patient, who has progressed to 8 cm, has developed a worrying CTG with variable decelerations and produced some meconium-stained liquor. She has had two uncomplicated deliveries in the past. Simultaneously, a patient on whom you are conducting an attempt at vaginal delivery after having had a caesarean section for her first child, has suddenly developed a very irregular fetal heart rate pattern.

What would you do and why?

Examiner's instructions

The candidate should recognize that all three situations pose risk to the life of mother or fetus or both: retained placenta leading to PPH in the first; fetal distress indicated by abnormal CTGs in the other two cases; and risk of scar rupture in the third case. The key here is to acquire information in order to prioritize and bring in help if feasible.

The following points should be discussed, and the marks awarded as indicated:

1. ***General impressions***: 5
   - Approach
   - Ability to prioritize
   - Ability to delegate
   - Problem solving
   - Decisiveness.
2. ***First case***: 5
   - Is she bleeding? — if not, reduces priority
   - are her obs stable?

- SHO/midwife to put up IV infusion. Start fluids
- Crossmatch blood — 2 units.

3. ***Second case*:** 5
   - Review CTG
   - Perform FBS unless CTG pathognomonic of fetal demise (from the description this is not the case)
   - Unless pH < 7.2 with high base excess, possibility of rapid progress to full dilatation and vaginal delivery.
4. ***Third case*:** 5
   - FHR abnormalities sensitive marker for scar complications
   - Look for corroborative features:

     — Poor progress/loss of uterine activity

     — PV bleeding

     — Uterine irregularity

     — Maternal tachycardia
   - Probably needs urgent delivery.
5. ***Prioritization and action*:** 5
   - Inform consultant and ask for help
   - Advise anaesthetic registrar to do likewise
   - Case 3: highest priority — on confirmation of abnormal CTG proceed to emergency laparotomy/caesarean section
   - Case 2: SHO or consultant to perform FBS
   - Case 1: if not bleeding, could wait; if bleeding, could have manual removal by consultant in delivery room
   - Other permutations could be put forward with alternative circumstances — mark according to reasons given.

Total mark out of 25: divide by 2.5 for final mark and round down part of mark

STATION 5.6

Shoulder dystocia: neonatal management

Marks

Candidate's instructions

You are called to an unexpected case of shoulder dystocia on the labour ward. When you deliver the baby he is pale, motionless and apnoeic. The mother is fine and is not bleeding. The paediatrician has been called but has not yet arrived. Summarize your actions for the examiner.

Examiner's instructions

The following should be discussed and marked as indicated:

- The baby is white, flaccid and apnoeic: he is likely to have experienced a severe acute hypoxic event during cord occlusion. Call for a resuscitaire (heat source, oxygen, suction, etc.), if not already in room. Clamp the cord, ask the midwife to supervise the mother while you attend to the baby and arrange for the paediatrician to be emergency-bleeped. **4**
- Dry the baby with a (warm) towel and keep him warm. **1**
- Assess him while administering facial oxygen and allocate an Apgar score (1 minute). **1**
- Ensure that the airway is clear, position the baby face-upwards with the head supported in a neutral position. **1**
- If respiratory effort is shallow or still absent, stimulate gently and offer supplementary oxygen. **1**
- Assess heart rate (stethoscope or feel pulsation at base of cord). If heart rate is less than 100 beats per minute or is decreasing, start lung inflation with 100% oxygen by mask. **1**
- Apply the mask over nose and mouth, holding the chin gently forward. Squeeze resuscitation bag slowly with finger tips at rate of 30–40 breaths per minute. See that the chest wall moves with inflations. Listen for breath and heart sounds. **2**
- If there is no prompt response and the heart rate is falling, ensure that the equipment is connected and oxygen functional. Call again for help. **2**
- Ask midwife or available person to continue ventilation. Administer external cardiac massage: external chest

compression is achieved by applying pressure with two fingers over the lower third of the sternum or by placing the thumbs over the lower third of the sternum with the hands around the chest. Compress by only 2–3 cm each time, at a rate of two compressions per second. Reinflate lungs after every three compressions. **2**

- After resuscitation, or when other staff have arrived, inform parents of what has happened and the actions you have taken. Document your actions in the case records. **1**
- Experienced resuscitators should attempt endotracheal intubation if Apgar score is 3 or less at or after 1 minute. Unless the operator is skilled in this technique, however, bag and mask ventilation is more effective. **1**
- If the heart rate does not respond, drugs and fluids will be given (via umbilical vein). Consider hypovolaemia or possibility of acute blood loss. **1**
- Naloxone is not a resuscitative drug but is given to an apnoeic baby whose mother has received opiates 2–4 hours previously — *after* adequate resuscitation. **2**

Total mark out of 20; divide by 2 for final mark

STATION 5.7
Colposcopy — role-play

Candidate's instructions

You are the doctor carrying out the colposcopy clinic. Mrs Simpson (age 45) has been referred to your colposcopy clinic because a routine cervical smear has been reported as showing CIN3 and she is very worried.

The clinic has a policy of sending out information to the patient prior to her visit. It normally uses a 'see and treat' policy, using LLETZ (large loop excision of the transformation zone).

How would you manage this situation, and advise this patient?

Role-player's instructions

You are 45 and married and you have been told by your GP that your smear shows 'CIN3'. You are unsure what this means, and the GP did not explain, just saying that you needed a colposcopy examination. You are worried. You received and read the information sheet but you do not really understand what it means.

If you do not get adequate explanations, express your concern about the following issues:

- *Is it cancer?*
- *How did I get it? Can I infect someone else?*
- *What is colposcopy?*
- *What is the treatment?*
- *Will it hurt?*
- *How effective is the treatment?*
- *Does the treatment have after-effects?*
- *Will I be told the results of the tests?*
- *How will I know that it has been cleared up?*
- *Will it come back?*

Examiner's instructions

This is a counselling station which assess the candidate's ability to explain the technique of colposcopy — carefully, in plain language and sympathetically — in a way which will gain the patient's confidence. The candidate will be judged on her ability to communicate with the patient. The following should be assessed and marked as shown:

- Greets the patient and introduces him/herself 1
- Asks if the patient has read the information sheet and *assesses the patient's understanding* about the cytological smear report 1
- Builds on this knowledge and *explains CIN3*: 1

  — Not cancer

  — Precancerous condition, but has the potential to progress to cancer

  — Might reverse spontaneously but this is unlikely

  — Can be easily eliminated, with simple treatment, usually as an outpatient

  — Occasionally may require inpatient treatment

  Explains *aetiology* — 'How did I get it?' 1

  — Related to intercourse

  — Thought to be related to wart virus infection, among other aetiological factors

- Assesses the patient's knowledge about colposcopy, builds on this and *explains the procedure*: 1

  — Colposcope — a viewing device 'similar to binoculars' which allows examination of the surface of the cervix

  — Examines the pattern of the surface cells and blood vessels

  — Uses a speculum to expose the cervix (the colposcope does not enter the vagina)

- Explains the use of local anaesthetic and answers the question, *Will colposcopy hurt?* . . . 'No, the speculum will stretch or open the vagina and may be uncomfortable but it is not painful' 1
- Obtains *consent* 1
- Explains punch biopsy and *treatment*: 1

  — Explains LLETZ — removal of a piece of cervical tissue which can be examined by the pathologist. Explains the noise of the diathermy machine and smoke extractor

— If certain of the nature of the abnormality and if the whole lesion is visible, then it is possible to treat the area at this visit. May require second treatment

- Explains features of post-treatment *recovery*: 1

— Initial postoperative uterine cramps and discomfort, may need to use mild analgesics

— The treatment will cause a raw or healing surface – should avoid coitus, tampons etc. for 2–3 weeks

— She should expect a serosanguinous vaginal discharge

— Warn about signs of pelvic infection

— Advises patient to return to the unit if she is concerned

- Explains *follow-up*. 1

Total mark out of 10

STATION 5.8
Domestic violence

Candidate's instructions

The patient you are about to see is attending the hospital for a routine antenatal visit at 35 weeks gestation. Before you go to see her the midwife speaks to you outside the room. She is concerned about the patient, who is complaining of rather vague symptoms of headache and generalized aches and pains. She is not sleeping. She has several bruises on her body and is reluctant to explain how they came about.

You have 15 minutes to see this patient: advise her as you feel necessary, based on what you learn during your consultation.

Role-player's instructions

You are 22 years old, this is your third pregnancy, and you have reached 35 weeks. You booked at the maternity hospital at 12 weeks and you were last seen in the hospital at 18 weeks. You were supposed to be receiving shared antenatal care with your GP but have not attended the surgery.

There have been no complications with your pregnancy to date but you have been having domestic problems with your partner. You have been married to your partner, Simon, for three years. You first met him when you were 18 and became pregnant soon afterwards. Simon works as a garage mechanic. Recently he claims to have been under a lot of pressure at work and has been arriving home later and later. You moved to this area recently and have no family or friends who live nearby.

Soon after you were married he began to beat you. Since the beginning of this pregnancy the beatings have become more violent and more frequent and you no longer feel safe at home. You are also becoming concerned for the safety of the other two children. He returned home late last night, offering no explanation of where he had been. You argued and he beat you viciously. You now feel that you need help but don't know where to turn.

You are now attending the antenatal clinic in the hospital for the first time since early pregnancy. The midwife has noticed the bruising and you mentioned to her that you have had headaches and generalized pains and have trouble sleeping. She has gone to get the doctor.

The doctor believes this is a routine visit but should be suspicious about the bruising, as the midwife has specifically mentioned it to him. If he inquires about the bruising you should open up and discuss the true situation.

If, after a few minutes, the doctor makes no attempt to discuss the bruising you should initiate discussion about your domestic situation. Mention that you feel:

- Unable to cope with the violence
- Unsafe at home
- Concerned for the other children
- It is your fault
- Powerless, frightened of officialdom/agencies and fearful of the repercussions of disclosure.

Examiner's instructions

The following should be assessed and marked:

• Greeting and introduction	**1**
• Use of simple language, without medical jargon	**1**
• Eye contact	**1**
• Obtains personal details	**1**
• Current pregnancy (general details)	**1**
• Social/personal history	**1**
• Enquiries about bruising	**1**
• Sympathetic approach	**1**
• Ability to listen	**1**
• Relevance of direct questions	**1**
• Non-judgmental approach	**1**
• Emotional support	**1**
• Confidentiality (except Mental Health Order and child protection procedures)	**1**
• Relevance of advice:	
— remove from at-risk situation (stay with friends or relatives; refuge or temporary accommodation)	**1**
— social worker	**1**
— Women's Aid helpline	**1**
— legal options	**1**
• Awareness of where to get help — contact numbers	**1**
• Marks from role-player.	**2**

Total mark out of 20: divide by 2 for final mark

Notes

Management of domestic violence is always very difficult. In the situation portrayed the patient has reached the point were she realises that she is in need of help and is prepared to accept it. The attending staff must be aware that she is at considerable physical risk. It is also likely that her children are at risk.

It is important that the staff do not act in a judgmental fashion. They must act in such a manner as to protect the confidentiality of all concerned, except for the obligations that may arise from the Mental Health Act and child protection procedures.

The first step is to ensure that the mother and children are removed from the risk situation. In some situations this may be achieved within the family, but in this case the patient has no family and no local support and both mother and children may have to be taken into care.

It is important to involve the help of social workers and the social services agencies. Whether the woman will accept these services or not, it is important that she be made aware of the availability of help and how it can be accessed at any time (Helplines, refuge accommodation, helpgroups etc.).

STATION 5.9

Shoulder dystocia: obstetric management

Marks

Candidate's instructions

You are the registrar on call and you are 'crash-called' to a delivery room because of shoulder dystocia. Discuss your subsequent actions with the examiner.

Examiner's instructions

The following should be discussed and marked as indicated:

- Ensure paediatrician and anaesthetist have been called **4**
- Ensure enough assistants present (minimum of three) **2**
- Move mother into McRobert's position, if not already adopted (mother on back, femora abducted, rotated outwards and flexed, with maternal thighs to maternal abdomen — requires one assistant for each leg) **4**
- Take over delivery, ensuring large episiotomy is made **2**
- Ascertain position of fetal shoulders **2**
- Suprapubic pressure to be applied by an assistant, pushing the anterior shoulder forwards and down **3**
- Apply steady, but not excessive, traction to head and neck. **1**

This should be sufficient to deliver around 90% of cases. If there is failure to deliver, the following manoeuvres should be attempted, with anaesthetic assistance as appropriate.

- 'Woods screw' — hand inserted into the vagina and pressure applied to anterior aspect of the posterior shoulder in the direction of the fetal back, attempting to bring the shoulders into the oblique plane. Suprapubic pressure should then be used to bring the anterior shoulder into the pelvis, below the pubic bone **2**
- 'Reverse Woods screw' – rotation in the opposite direction. Some may opt to try rotation in this direction first **2**
- If these are unsuccessful, an attempt to deliver the posterior arm should be made. This involves reaching high enough posteriorly to flex the arm at the elbow and then sweep it across the chest and face. Some force may be required and fractures to the humerus or clavicle may be sustained. **2**

Failing this, measures of last resort are used:

- Deliberately breaking of the clavicles to reduce bisacromial diameter, either using pressure between finger and thumb, or using scissors **1**
- Cephalic replacement and caesarean section (Zaveanelli manoeuvre) **1**
- Symphysiotomy, using a urethral catheter to displace the urethra and dividing the anterior and inferior parts of the pubic symphysis by cutting *down* with a scalpel, towards the finger in the vagina. **1**

The candidate should be aware of the main *potential complications* of shoulder dystocia:

- Maternal soft-tissue trauma, including cervical tears, third-degree tears and massive haemorrhage and PPH **3**
- Stillbirth/neonatal death **1**
- Hypoxic ischaemic encephalopathy/cerebral palsy **1**
- Erb's palsy **1**
- Klumpke's palsy. **1**

General points:

- The candidate should be aware of the importance of accurately documenting the sequence of events in the notes **2**
- The simplest manoeuvres — McRobert's position, generous episiotomy and suprapubic pressure — should always be attempted *before* the more traumatic manoeuvres **2**
- Excessive force, and in particular, excessive downward traction on the fetal head and neck, should be avoided until all other manoeuvres have been attempted. **2**

Total mark out of 40: divide by 4 for final mark

STATION 5.10

Unexplained infertility

Marks

Candidate's instructions

Discuss with the examiner the different options available to a young couple (both age 25) with unexplained secondary infertility of 18 months duration.

Examiner's instructions

The following should be discussed and marks awarded as shown. If specific points are not mentioned by the candidate, the examiner should raise them to prompt the discussion:

- Expectant management (i.e. no treatment) for up to 3 years should be considered — results in pregnancy rates of up to 80%. 2
- There is no good evidence that clomifene will increase the pregnancy rate above that of expectant management. It will, however, lead to a 10% multiple pregnancy rate in these who become pregnant while taking it. 2
- Bromocriptine is not effective. 1
- Danazol is not effective and will probably act as a contraceptive. 1
- GIFT and IVF are both effective. 2
- IVF is preferable to GIFT as it provides diagnostic information about the ability of the sperm to fertilize the ovum and the quality of the embryos. In addition, it does not require laparoscopy. 2

Total mark out of 10

ORAL ASSESSMENT EXAMINATION

6

STATION 6.1

Cervical screening presentation — preparatory station

Candidate's instructions

At the next station you will be required to make a 15-minute presentation to General Practitioner (GP) trainees on the principles behind the NHS cervical cytological screening programme (NHSCSP). Your presentation should cover the value of the screening programme, the screening methods, and the incidence and management of cytological abnormalities.

You may use a maximum of three acetate sheets (A4 size) which will be provided.

STATION 6.2

Cervical screening presentation — examination station

Marks

Examiner's instructions

The presentation should cover the following points:

1. ***Why cervical screening?*** **2**
    - Reduces incidence of cervical carcinoma
    - Significant reduction in incidence of cervical carcinoma since 1987
    - No reduction in incidence of cervical carcinoma with *opportunistic* screening.
2. ***Who should be screened?*** **2**
    - Screening should target the total 'at risk' population: it should not be opportunistic
    - All sexually active women age 20–65
    - All women with a past history of cervical dysplasia and possibly other high-risk groups.
3. ***Who should* not *be screened?*** **2**
    - Age < 20
    - Age > 65 with three normal smears over previous 10 years
    - After hysterectomy, with normal smears over previous 10 years
    - Those who have *never* been sexually active.
4. **How to screen — cytological methods:** **2**
    - Cervical cytology — Papanicolaou's (Pap) smear
    - Must sample squamocolumnar junction (SCJ) and transformation zone
    - Difficulties may be encountered if there has been treatment to the cervix or in postmenopausal women
    - Ayers spatula — should be abandoned due to high incidence of poor quality smears
    - Aylesbury spatula extends into endocervical canal, improves quality of sampling
    - Cytobrush — useful for sampling the SCJ when this is high in endocervical canal.

5. ***How often to screen?*** 2

- One smear results in 70–80% sensitivity in detecting an abnormality
- Two smears result in 95% sensitivity in detecting an abnormality
- Frequency intervals: 3 years for NHSCSP; 1 year for Canada; and 5 years for UK (NHS) for economic reasons.

Total mark out of 10

STATION 6.3

Previous caesarean section

Marks

Candidate's instructions

In your antenatal clinic you have a 28-year-old patient in her third pregnancy, at 42 weeks gestation. Her first baby was delivered vaginally without any problem. Her second pregnancy was complicated by placenta praevia and her baby was delivered by elective caesarean section without complications. Her pregnancy so far has been uncomplicated, the fetus has grown normally and is presenting cephalically with the head three-fifths palpable.

Describe your management and how you would counsel the patient.

Examiner's instructions

Notes

- The candidate should be aware of postmaturity
- He should know that vaginal delivery rate in these circumstances is in the region of 75–80%
- Caesarean section would increase maternal morbidity and mortality
- Induction of labour in women who have had a previous caesarean section is well documented and does not appear to significantly increase the risk of scar complication though care must be exercised
- Careful clinical assessment must be performed
- There has to be sensitive and skilful counselling
- Clinical management must be clearly and carefully planned.

Keeping these points in mind, the candidate should be assessed and marked as follows:

1. **Immediate appraisal — *What is your assessment of the situation?***
   - She is postmature 1
   - Normally, induction of labour and delivery *would* be undertaken 1
   - Her chances of successful vaginal delivery are of the order of 75–80% 1

- Repeat CS increases maternal morbidity and mortality when compared with vaginal delivery but there is a *20–25% chance of emergency CS.* **1**

2. **Options for delivery — *What are your clinical options, assuming assessments of mother and fetus do not indicate compromise?***
   - Conservative management in anticipation of spontaneous labour, and careful fetal monitoring (although this is not of proven efficacy) **1**
   - Induction of labour: **1**
     - — Scar complication rate no greater than with spontaneous labour **1**
     - — CESDI warning about repeated doses of vaginal prostaglandins and perinatal deaths **1**
   - Elective caesarean section. **1**

3. **Clinical Assessment — *What clinical factors would you take into account?***
   - General well-being of mother and fetus **1**
   - Possibility of placenta praevia and/or implantation of placenta over previous uterine scar (placenta accreta/percreta ⇒ weakened scar) **1**
   - Bishop score/cervical assessment **1**
   - Maternal wishes. **1**

4. **Counselling — *The baby is an average size and, clinically, there appears to be adequate liquor. Fetal activity is good. The Bishop Score is 8/13. How would you counsel the patient ?***
   - Explain current situation and options **1**
   - Explain procedures for induction of labour and rationale behind each method **1**
   - Amniotomy and oxytocin infusion appropriate. Vaginal prostaglandins an alternative **1**
   - If vaginal PGE_2 is used, give no more than one 1 mg dose **1**
   - 75–80% chance of vaginal delivery if labour is spontaneous — a little lower than this with induction (favourable cervix) **1**
   - Up to 1% risk of scar complication — serious, therefore close monitoring in labour and lower threshold for caesarean section **1**
   - Seek mother's views and wishes. **1**

Total mark out of 20: divide by 2 for final mark

STATION 6.4

Exposure to rubella

Marks

Candidate's instructions

A 25-year-old woman attends the booking clinic. She is 7 weeks pregnant and informs you that 5 days previously she went to visit her sister. Three days after the visit her sister rang her to say that her son (the patient's nephew) had developed a rash and the GP had diagnosed German measles. The patient checked with her mother and was told that she had had German measles as a child, and so was reassured.

What would your management be?

Examiner's instructions

The following points should be covered, and marks allocated accordingly. If a point is not mentioned by the candidate, the examiner should ask specifically about it:

- Many viral illnesses produce a rubella-like clinical picture. A history of rubella should not therefore be accepted without serological evidence of previous infection: she should have blood samples taken to check for rubella IgG. **4**
- The period of infectivity is from 1 week before until 4 days after the onset of the rash. The nephew in this case was, therefore, infectious. **2**
- The risk of congenital rubella syndrome (CRS) is up to 90% if the infection is contracted within the first 10 weeks of pregnancy. The patient here is at maximum risk. **2**
- CRS can lead to mental handicap, cataract, deafness, cardiac abnormalities, inflammatory lesions of the brain, liver, lungs and bone-marrow, and IUGR. **4**

The patient was found to be non-immune — What is the next step?

- The nephew may not have had rubella. He should have his infection status assessed by saliva sample, checked for rubella IgM. Blood samples could be taken, but saliva collection is less invasive. **2**

The nephew had confirmed rubella. — What should be done next?

- The patient should have further blood samples taken 21 days after exposure to confirm if she contracted rubella. The timing is important because the incubation period is 14–21 days. **2**

The patient did not contract rubella. What should you do next?

- Reassurance **1**
- Postnatal rubella vaccination. **3**

Total mark out of 20: divide by 2 for final mark

STATION 6.5	
Genital herpes in pregnancy	Marks

Candidate's instructions

You have received the following GP letter:

> Dear Colleague,
>
> Please could you review this primigravid patient who is booked under your care. She is currently 37 weeks gestation and appears to have genital herpes.
>
> Yours sincerely,

Discuss with the examiner how you would manage this patient.

Examiner's instructions

The following points should be discussed, and marks awarded as indicated:

1. ***Arrange to review the patient that week.*** 1
2. ***History***
   - Primary or secondary attack? 1
   - Duration of attack 1
   - Symptoms (pain, dysuria, difficulty voiding) 1
   - Sexual contacts. 1
3. ***Examination***
   - Inspect for characteristic lesions (vesicles — viral swab if in doubt) 1
   - Look for secondary bacterial infection 1
   - Speculum examination. 1
4. ***Investigations***
   - Triple swabs (for PID) plus pus swab if indicated 1
   - HIV testing 1
   - Screening of partner(s) — involve GUM clinic. 1

5. ***Treatment***

- Aciclovir: usually oral; IV if unwell (unlicensed but appears safe, most effective if used early in attack) **3**
- Lignocaine gel (for pain) **1**
- Antibiotics for secondary bacterial infection **1**
- Advice regarding voiding urine (PU in bath, catheter if in retention). **1**

6. ***Counselling***

- Advice regarding sexual transmission **1**
- Possibility of other STDs, hence swabs +/– HIV test **1**
- Risk to baby from other STDs **1**
- Risk to baby from herpes (minimal if secondary, significant if primary) **1**
- Aim to allow vaginal delivery if no active lesions in labour. **2**
- If active lesions: caesarean section **2**
- Inform paediatricians (urine and stool samples and surface swabs from infant if risk of infection) **1**
- Prophylactic treatment of neonate if risk of infection significant. **1**

7. ***Risks***

- Neonatal herpes rare in UK (1.65 / 100 000) **1**
- Risk of vertical transmission with *primary infection in third trimester and vaginal delivery — around* 40% **1**
- Risk of transmission with active secondary infection in labour and vaginal delivery—1 to 4%. **1**

Total mark out of 30: divide by 3 for final mark

STATION 6.6

Neonatal survival at 28 weeks

Marks

Candidate's instructions

An anxious pregnant woman, whose fetus shows severe IUGR at 28 weeks gestation, wishes to know about the outlook for her baby should she be delivered soon. Discuss with the examiner what information you would offer this patient about her baby.

Examiner's instructions

The following points should be discussed and marks awarded as shown below:

- In general, neonatal survival rates at this gestation are over 90%. 1
- If gestation can be prolonged, however, the probability of survival increases and the likelihood that the baby will need intensive care diminishes (50% at 30 weeks). Therefore prolongation of pregnancy is desirable. 1
- Fetal wellbeing can be monitored regularly (growth, BPP) to ensure that prolongation of pregnancy is not compromising the baby. 1
- Neonatal survival can be optimized by administering prenatal steroids (which will be done if those caring for her feel that she is likely to be delivered within 7 days). 1
- Delivery should take place in a centre with neonatal intensive care facilities and in optimal conditions. 1
- Neonatal course is likely to include respiratory distress syndrome — requiring surfactant administration and respiratory support (CPAP or ventilation) and oxygen administration thereafter. Other possible neonatal problems include vulnerability to infection, jaundice requiring phototherapy; the possible need for IV nutrition, patent ductus arteriosus; and brain problems (intraventricular haemorrhage or periventricular leucomalacia). The incidence of such brain problems is less than 10% at this gestation. 3
- The baby will be in hospital for several months — average discharge time is around the due date — thereafter requiring outpatient follow-up with screening of vision, hearing, growth and neurological development. 1

- The mother can express breast milk for her baby until he is able to suckle, at the time approximately equivalent to 34 weeks gestation. 1

Total mark out of 10

STATION 6.7

Thromboembolic prophylaxis in gynaecological surgery — preparatory station

This is a preparatory station. You are asked to design a protocol for risk assessment and prophylaxis for thromboembolic disease in gynaecological surgery in your hospital. You will be asked to discuss your protocol with the examiner in the next station.

STATION 6.8

Thromboembolic prophylaxis in gynaecological surgery — examination station Marks

Examiner's instructions

The candidate will present her protocol and the following points should be discussed, and marked as shown:

- *Importance*: Thromboembolic disease (TED) is a major cause of mortality and morbidity in gynaecological surgery. For example, deep vein thrombosis (DVT) has a 12% prevalence following abdominal hysterectomy and TED accounts for about 20% of perioperative deaths. **5**
- *Risk Assessment*: Cases should be divided into different categories according to their risk and the type of prophylactic measures required. **2**
- *Low risk*: includes minor surgery (< 30 minutes) with no other risk factors, major surgery (> 30 minutes), less than 40 years old with no other risk factors. TED prophylaxis — early ambulation and adequate hydration should be ensured. **5**
- *Moderate risk*: includes minor surgery (< 30 minutes) with a personal or family history of TED or thrombophilias, major surgery (> 30 minutes) with obesity (> 80 kg), gross varicose veins, current infection, heart failure, recent MI, major current illness, or preoperative immobility for more than 4 days. Prophylactic S/C unfractionated heparin 5000 iu (started 2 hours preoperatively and continued 12-hourly until discharge) with graduated elastic compression stockings should be used (in addition to early ambulation and adequate hydration) for TED prophylaxis. **5**
- *High risk*: includes any patient with three or more of the above mentioned risk factors, cancer surgery, and major surgery (>30 minutes) with a personal or family history of TED or thrombophilias. Prophylaxis is as for moderate risk but heparin should be started 12 hours preoperatively and be given 8-hourly until discharge. **5**
- *Effectiveness*: These measures will reduce the incidence of TED by two-thirds. **2**
- *Side-effects*:
  - — prophylactic heparin may lead to a 5–15% increase in wound haematoma. This is reduced by administering it well away from the wound (i.e. flank or thigh). **2**

— prophylactic heparin may lead to thrombocytopenia. Check platelet count if heparin used for more than 5 days. The use of low-molecular-weight heparin is an alternative and may reduce this risk. 2

- *Logistics*: the protocol should indicate who should perform the risk assessment and who should prescribe the heparin — the doctor listing the patient for surgery (i.e. in the clinic), the admitting officer, the surgeon or the anaesthetist. 2

Total mark out of 30: divide by 3 for final mark

STATION 6.9

Three clinical scenarios

Marks

Candidate's instructions

Your first-year SHO is just two weeks into the job and wishes to ask you some questions about clinical situations he has come across:

1. He has seen several ERPCs now and is concerned about the risk of uterine perforation. What should he tell the patients when obtaining their consent? How would he know if he had perforated the uterus and how could he prevent it happening? How do you manage a perforation?
2. A patient he has seen in the clinic with menorrhagia has asked him about endometrial ablation. She is coming in for hysteroscopy and curettage. What does endometrial resection involve and what should he tell her?
3. He has seen one of your colleagues perform an open salpingectomy for an ectopic pregnancy. He thought ectopic pregnancies were all done laparoscopically with conservation of the tubes.

Examiner's instructions

The following features of the three scenarios should be discussed and marked as shown:

1. ***Uterine perforation***

- All patients should be warned that there is a small (less than 1%) risk of perforation. **1**
- If the uterus is perforated, antibiotics and an overnight stay will be necessary. **1**
- Usually a laparoscopy will be performed to check for internal bleeding and allow the procedure to be completed under direct vision. Occasionally, if there is bleeding or concern about visceral injury, a laparotomy may be required. **2**
- The way to avoid perforation is good technique and the SHO should not be performing ERPCs unsupervised until he has been assessed as competent. **2**
- Perforation is more likely if the cervix is stenosed, in later gestations and in the presence of infection. More senior staff should be involved in these circumstances. **1**

- Perforation should be suspected if an instrument is inserted fully without encountering resistance. **1**
- A uterine dilator is blunt and unlikely to cause visceral damage. Senior assistance should be called and the procedure completed under laparoscopic control. **1**
- If forceps are opened through the perforation, or a curette used through the perforation, a laparotomy may be necessary in order to inspect the bowel. **1**

2. ***Endometrial resection***

- Endometrial resection is a procedure designed to *permanently* destroy the endometrium, hence stopping menstruation. **1**
- The procedure is likely to render the woman infertile, but she should continue to use reliable contraception since a pregnancy would be dangerous (risk of placenta accreta). **1**
- There may still be some menstrual loss following the procedure but, overall, 80% of women are happy with the result at one year. Long-term satisfaction may be less than this. **2**
- The procedure is traditionally carried out under hysteroscopic control with a general anaesthetic. It is usually a day-case procedure taking 20–30 minutes. **1**
- It is not suitable for women whose endometrial cavity is significantly distorted by fibroids and endometrial cancer must be excluded first. **1**
- There is a small risk of uterine perforation (around 1%). This may lead to the procedure being abandoned. **1**
- There is a very small risk of major haemorrhage or bowel damage following perforation. This could lead to a laparotomy. **1**
- Other methods are being developed (e.g. thermal ablation, microwave ablation) which may be quicker and safer. **1**
- Mirena should be considered. **1**

3. ***Surgical management of ectopic pregnancy***

- Laparotomy would have been indicated if the patient was shocked. **2**
- Laparotomy would have been indicated following laparoscopy if the surgeon did not have the skills to proceed laparoscopically. **1**

- If a tubal ectopic has ruptured a salpingectomy will usually be required in order to stop the bleeding. 1
- Even if a tubal ectopic has not ruptured, a salpingectomy is currently recommended in cases where the contralateral tube appears healthy. 1
- This is because subsequent pregnancy rates appear to be comparable, and removing the tube reduces the risk of complications. 1
- Complications of salpingostomy include persistent trophoblast and an increased risk of recurrent ectopic pregnancy in the damaged tube. 2
- Salpingostomy requires follow-up with serial HCGs and persistent trophoblast may require treatment with methotrexate or further surgery. 1
- Where possible this should be discussed with the patient prior to surgery. 1

Total mark out of 30: divide by 3 for final mark

STATION 6.10	
Breech presentation — role-play	Marks

Candidate's instructions

Mrs Smith is a 28-year-old primigravida who now is at 35 weeks of gestation and is found to have a breech presentation.

How would you advise her?

Role-player's instructions

You are 35 weeks pregnant and your baby is 'breech'. You are concerned about the position of the baby and want to know what your choices are.

The doctor should ask you a series of questions about your height (155 cm), blood group (O Rh-negative) and whether you have had any previous bleeding (no). You have no other medical conditions.

The doctor should suggest trying to 'turn the baby' or external cephalic version (ECV) — you are concerned about the safety of the suggested procedure.

The procedure is carried out but is unsuccessful. You wish to know how the baby will be delivered and if vaginal breech delivery is safe.

Examiner's instructions

The following points should be discussed and marked as indicated:

	Marks
• Ability to develop rapport with patient	2
• Explanation to patient	2
• Elicits history of contraindications to ECV (none relevant, except Rhesus-negative)	2
• Explanation of procedure:	
— Manipulation	1
— USS control	1
— Anti-D prophylaxis	1
• Safety — no evidence of increased risk	2
• Reduces risk of CS by about 50%.	2

Inform the candidate that the procedure was unsuccessful.The role player asks: "*How will my baby be delivered now? Is vaginal deliver safe?*"

- Explains that planned caesarean section is safer than vaginal delivery as it has been shown to reduce the likelihood of perinatal mortality, neonatal mortality or serious neonatal morbidity by two-thirds (relative risk 0.33) with no increase in maternal mortality or serious maternal morbidity. **7**

Total mark out of 20: divide by 2 for final mark

ORAL ASSESSMENT EXAMINATION

7

STATION 7.1

Exposure to chickenpox in pregnancy

Marks

Candidate's instructions

A 23-year-old pregnant woman at 12 weeks gestation had been visited by her sister and 5-year-old nephew 2 days ago. Her sister rang her last night to tell her that her nephew had developed chickenpox. She does not remember having the infection as a child. She went to her GP for advice and he rang you. *What advice would you give and why?*

Examiner's instructions

The following points should be covered, and marks allocated as shown:

- The infectivity period starts 2 days before appearance of the rash (and lasts until the vesicles are dry). Therefore the nephew was infective when he came in contact with the patient. **1**
- Despite the absence of a history of previous exposure, the patient has an 85% chance of being immune. She should have blood taken and tested for varicella antibodies (IgG). If she is found to be immune, no action is needed. **1**
- Until her varicella status is sorted out, the patient should be advised not to come in contact with pregnant women, in case she is infective. She should *not* come to the antenatal clinic during this time. **1**
- If she is found to be non-immune, she should be given varicella-zoster immunoglobulins (VZIG) as soon as is practically possible. VZIG will prevent or attenuate maternal/fetal varicella infection if given up to 10 days after exposure. **2**
- Detection of VZ IgM in maternal serum indicates primary VZ infection. Occuring in the first 20 weeks of pregnancy, primary infection carries a 2% risk of congenital varicella infection (includes skin scarring, eye defects, hyperplasia of limbs, neurological abnormalities). Referral to a specialist centre for detailed ultrasound scan at 16 weeks gestation or 5 weeks after infection, whichever is sooner, should be considered. **2**
- Neonatal ophthalmic examination should be organized at birth. **1**

- Maternal varicella infection (at any stage of pregnancy) carries the risk of maternal varicella pneumonia, which complicates up to 10% of cases and has a mortality rate of up to 30%. Treatment is with parenteral aciclovir. 2

Total mark out of 10

STATION 7.2	
Rubella immunization	Marks

Candidate's instructions

A 23-year-old pregnant woman was found to be non-immune to rubella at booking. She has now had a caesarean delivery and you are seeing her on day 3 postoperatively to advise about rubella immunization.

Examiner's and role-player's instructions

The following points should be covered, and marked as shown:

- Introduction (name and grade) 1
- Puts patient at ease 1
- Explains the condition and intended action 1
- Avoidance of medical jargon 1
- Appropriate eye contact 1
- Invites questions and listens attentively. 1

The role-player will ask the following questions:

What type of vaccine is this?

- Weak virus (live attenuated). 1

Does this mean that I should not get pregnant after taking it?

- Yes, but only avoid pregnancy for 1 month. 1

Does this also mean that I should not be in contact with pregnant women?

- No it does not. There is no risk of infection to pregnant women from contact with recently immunized individuals. 1

I have received a blood transfusion at my caesarean section. Does that make any difference to the rubella immunization?

- Yes. Blood transfusion inhibits the response in up to 50% of rubella vaccination. In such cases a test for antibody should be performed 8 weeks later, with re-immunization if necessary. 1

Total mark out of 10

STATION 7.3

Counselling for sterilization

Marks

Candidate's instructions

A 35-year-old woman has requested sterilization. She has four children, is in a stable relationship and both she and her husband are sure that they have completed their family. They currently use the male condom for contraception. She has a BMI of 25 and has had no previous operations. *What information would you give her about the sterilization?*

Examiner's instructions

The following should be discussed, and marks allocated as shown:

- Other methods of birth control, including male sterilization. **4**
- The risks of laparoscopy (bowel, bladder and blood vessel injury) and the chance of requiring laparotomy if problems are encountered (1–2 per 1000). **4**
- The method of access (laparoscopy) and tubal occlusion (e.g. Filshie clips) that you would recommend in her case and the method that would be used if this intended method fails for any reason (e.g. laparotomy if laparoscopy is not possible). **4**
- The associated failure rate (approximately 1 in 200) and the fact that pregnancies can occur several years after the procedure. **2**
- If the sterilization fails, the resulting pregnancy may be ectopic and the patient should seek medical advice if she thinks (at any time following the sterilization) that she might be pregnant or if she has abnormal abdominal pain or vaginal bleeding. **4**
- Reassurance that tubal occlusion is not associated with an increased risk of heavier or irregular periods. **2**
- Advice to continue the use of contraception until the menstrual period following the procedure. It should be explained, however, that the sterilization procedure does not guard against pregnancy that may have occurred before the procedure (despite contraception) and may be undetectable (too early). **4**
- Explanation that the procedure is intended to be permanent. **4**
- Explanation should also be given about the success rate associated with reversal and its availability, should this be

necessary in the future. The success rate depends on the method used for sterilization (e.g. Filshie clips versus diathermy) and the availability of local expertise in microsurgery. 2

Total mark out of 30: divide by 3 for final mark

Notes

The explanation about reversibility is a contentious issue. Many gynaecologists are of the view that if it is mentioned by the patient or doctor this implies lack of commitment to the intended permanence of the sterilization. However, many patients already know about it and a body of literature exists dealing with it. In addition, the RCOG in its *Clinical Guidelines* (1999) recommends giving this information to the patient.

STATION 7.4

Aetiology of cerebral palsy

Candidate's instructions

You are a consultant obstetrician and have received the following letter from your paediatric colleague:

> Dear Mr Jones,
>
> Re: Baby Wallace — age 8 months
>
> Please will you see the parents of this baby at their request. I have been following up baby Wallace since birth because of his low birth weight. When I saw him this time he was still not sitting independently and on examination his legs are stiff, with exaggerated deep tendon reflexes. I have had to tell his parents that I suspect he has cerebral palsy.
>
> Unfortunately, they have become very angry and are thinking of filing a complaint about their baby's delivery. They are blaming the condition on delay in performing the caesarean section.
>
> As you will recall, this lady is a 28-year-old multipara, a heavy smoker with mild essential hypertension. She had an uneventful pregnancy until 34 weeks when, because of concern about fundal height, she had an ultrasound scan. This revealed a symmetrically small baby on the 10th centile. Fetal parameters were otherwise good and the liquor volume was normal. Repeat ultrasound scan two weeks later showed some growth and adequate liquor. She was admitted in early labour at 37 weeks. CTG showed occasional variable decelerations although the baseline heart rate was normal and reactive, and you performed a caesarean section 1 hour later (because she had had two previous sections).
>
> This baby was in excellent condition at birth, with Apgar scores of 9 and 10 and normal cord pH, but weighed only 1.8 kg which was below the 2nd centile. He was not obviously dysmorphic and behaved normally postnatally. He was discharged home at 4 days, bottle-feeding well.
>
> Thank you for agreeing to see these parents.
>
> Yours sincerely
>
> Dr Carson
> Consultant Paediatrician

Role-player's instructions

Your 8-month old baby has cerebral palsy. During the pregnancy it was found, at 34 weeks, that the baby was smaller than expected. Monitoring tests were normal and you came into hospital in labour at 37 weeks. The baby's heart trace was not entirely normal and you had a caesarean section 1 hour after admission. The baby was born in a good condition, weighing 1.8 kg. However, he did not develop as expected and you went to see the paediatrician who told you that the baby probably has cerebral palsy.

You are very angry because you believe that the cerebral palsy was caused by the delay in delivery. You are seeing the obstetrician who was in charge of your pregnancy so that you can express your anger and make a complaint. You specifically want to ask why the baby was not delivered at 34 weeks when the problem was first detected and why he was not delivered *immediately*, when you were admitted in labour. You believe that both these delays were responsible for the cerebral palsy.

Examiner's instructions

The following points should be covered, and marked as indicated:

- Introduction and putting patient at ease **1**
- Listens calmly **1**
- Answers the questions **4**
- Uses plain English **1**
- Appropriate eye contact **1**
- Ability to defuse stress/anger. **1**

Role-player's assessment:

- Confidence in candidate. **1**

Total mark out of 10

Notes

The baby is likely to have spastic diplegia related to IUGR. It has only become obvious clinically at this age as the motor milestones are delayed due to the effects of unbalanced muscle tone. There is no suggestion that there was acute hypoxia prior to delivery or neonatal encephalopathy, to support a diagnosis of an acute intrapartum event. Earlier delivery, at 34 weeks, would have introduced avoidable complications of prematurity and would probably not have affected the eventual outcome.

The condition is related to interference with the normal development of periventricular white matter in the immature brain. This can be caused by chronic hypoxia/ischaemia, by reduced local perfusion or by metabolic factors (cytokines, interleukins) which are currently not measurable in clinical practice.

STATION 7.5

Preterm labour: in-utero transfer

Marks

Candidate's instructions

A 39-year-old patient has been admitted to the delivery suite with abdominal pains. These have been present for the last 2 hours. The pregnancy is at 32 weeks gestation. Clinically, the uterus is equivalent to dates. There is a cephalic presentation with the head engaged. Contractions can be palpated 2:10 minutes. Fetal heart rate recording is normal.

The pregnancy was conceived by IVF at the fifth attempt.

Your neonatal intensive care unit is full. The nearest cot is 3 hours travelling time away. Discuss your options with your consultant (the examiner).

Examiner's instructions

The candidate should establish the diagnosis; consider the options; evaluate the pros and cons of these options; and understand the needs of a neonate delivered at this gestation. The discussion should be marked as follows:

The candidate should first establish the diagnosis

- Confirm the clinical diagnosis (premature labour) 1
- Check for other causes of abdominal pain:
  - — Abruption 1
  - — UTI 1
  - — Appendicitis 1
- Perform a vaginal examination to assess cervical change. 1

The candidate is told that the cervix is 4 cm dilated, the head is just above the spines and the membranes are intact — ***What is your diagnosis and what are your concerns?***

- In premature labour 1
- Delivery imminent 1
- 'Precious' baby—increases maternal anxiety 1
- Steroids have not been administered and likelihood of less than 12 hours for them to act 1
- No neonatal cots available. 1

What are your options? Which would you opt for and why?

- Give steroids 1
- Tocolysis. May not be effective at this stage 1
- In-utero transfer to nearest unit with a cot. May deliver in transit 1
- Deliver in-house and transfer ex-utero — considerations include: 1
  - — Reported results indicate poorer outcome than in-utero transfer
  - — Paediatrician and neonatal nurse would have to travel with neonate — may not have staff to provide this support
  - — Receiving unit may have a retrieval system which could collect the neonate
- In-house delivery with ex-utero transfer may be the safest option. 1

If you were the only attendant at the delivery of this baby in non-ideal circumstances (e.g. in an ambulance en route to the receiving hospital) what would you do for the baby and why?

- Dry the baby 1
- Keep the baby warm (place between mother's breasts) 2
- Maintain oxygenation — mask — intubation as last resort. 2

Total mark out of 20: divide by 2 for final mark

STATION 7.6

Labour management

Marks

Candidate's instructions

As part of clinical governance you are asked to ensure that your caesarean section rate is in line with good practice. *How would you go about this?*

Examiner's instructions

Candidates should be aware that there is *no guidance regarding a specific rate*: this will be affected by case mix and complexity. They should also be aware that rates are rising. Most professional bodies have some concern over this, given the documented evidence of increased short-term morbidity and mortality rates associated with caesarean section.

The following should be discussed, and marks allocated as shown:

1. ***Awareness that caesarean section rates are rising and the consequences of this.*** **1**
2. ***Main causes*:** **2**
   - Failure to progress
   - Previous caesarean section
   - Fetal distress
   - Breech presentation.
3. ***Pre-labour measures*:**
   - ECV offered for breech presentation **1**
   - Pre-labour education of the mother. **1**
4. ***Labour management*:**
   - One-to-one midwifery **1**
   - Support during labour **1**
   - Correct diagnosis of labour **1**
   - Appropriate design and use of cervicogram/partogram **1**
   - Correct oxytocin dosages (30-minute increments) **1**
   - Low risk cases — no routine amniotomy or continuous electronic fetal monitoring **2**
   - pH measurement to back up CTG monitoring. **1**

5. ***Organisational issues*:**

- Consultant responsible for delivery suite **1**
- Formation of a 'delivery suite forum' (multidisciplinary) **1**
- Multidisciplinary educational programme **1**
- Supervision of juniors by seniors **1**
- Agreed policies and review procedures **1**
- Audit of policies and standards. **1**

6. ***Attempt at vaginal delivery for previous lower segment caesarean delivery.*** **1**

Total mark out of 20: divide by 2 for final mark

STATION 7.7

Patient request for caesarean section — role-play

Candidate's instructions

This patient requests an elective caesarean delivery. She is a 26-year-old paediatrician in her first pregnancy. She is fit and healthy and the pregnancy to date has been normal. The pregnancy is now 36 weeks advanced, fetal growth is normal, and the fetus presents cephalically with the head two-fifths palpable. You are required to counsel her.

Role-player's instructions

You are a 26-year-old paediatrician in your first pregnancy. You are fit and healthy and the pregnancy to date has been normal. You are now 36 weeks pregnant. The fetus has grown well and presents cephalically with the head two-fifths palpable. You do not want to go through the pain and uncertainty of a vaginal delivery (for yourself and your baby). You are also aware of the perineal damage which can result from a vaginal delivery and would prefer to accept the distinct, but very small, risks of an elective caesarean section. You do not plan to have more than two children and may consider sterilization after the second.

You should be firm and resolute in your request. You know that caesarean section removes the hypoxic 'stress' that labour normally causes the fetus and that birth trauma is reduced. You are also aware of the potential long-term morbidity of vaginal delivery in terms of urinary incontinence, prolapse and colorectal symptoms.

The candidate will almost certainly stress the risk of caesarean section — this should be challenged by asking: *Is there greater risk from an emergency section than from an elective section?* The candidate should agree that there is. Then ask: *Can you guarantee me a vaginal delivery?* to which the answer has to be 'No'. Then ask: '*So what is the risk on an 'intention to treat' basis of vaginal versus elective caesarean?*

If, on the other hand, the candidate offers no objection to your request, press him to explain the risks of caesarean section for yourself and your baby in a more even-handed way, then introduce the questions above.

Examiner's instructions

Notes: This is a challenging situation, both in real life and in the exam. However, it is an increasingly common situation. The candidate should know that there is an increased maternal mortality associated with caesarean delivery — hence the pressure from a number of quarters to keep the rate down. When fetal complications and morbidity from vaginal delivery are taken into account, however, the equation is more complicated and more evenly balanced. Analysis to date has often been simplistic and has often not taken into account intention-to-treat. Thus if emergency caesarean section rates rise due to failure to achieve vaginal delivery, the increased risk of emergency caesarean section will, to some extent, account for the lower risk quoted for straightforward elective section. The effects of caesarean section on future pregnancy are becoming clearer, particularly the increased risk of placenta praevia.

The following should be discussed, and marks allocated as indicated:

1. ***General assessment*** (these marks are allocated by the role-player): **5**
   - Introduction
   - Eye contact and appropriate use of language
   - Listening and summarizing.
2. ***Risk to maternal wellbeing from caesarean section*:** **5**
   - Increased maternal mortality: x5–6 over spontaneous vaginal delivery and × 3 on an intention-to-treat basis
   - Haemorrhage
   - Infection
   - Thromboembolism
   - Anaesthetic complications.
3. ***Increase in morbidity*:** **5**
   - Longer hospital stay (therefore increased use of resources)
   - Reduced fertility
   - Anaemia (increased likelihood of transfusion)
   - Wound infection.
4. ***Risks for subsequent pregnancy from caesarean section*:** **5**
   - Placenta praevia increased x4 after first section; x7 after second
   - Morbid adherence of the placenta
   - Increases need for caesarean delivery in future (may not be a major consideration with this patient)
   - Scar complication (very low for lower segment scar).

5. ***Risks to the fetus from caesarean section*:** **2**

- Iatrogenic prematurity
- Transient tachypnoea of the newborn.

6. ***Advantages of vaginal delivery*:** **3**

- Least short-term morbidity and mortality for the mother
- Minimal risk for future reproductive function
- Shorter hospital stay and quicker recovery
- Allows perinatal adaptation of the fetus to extrauterine existence.

7. ***Advantages of elective caesarean section*:** **5**

- Predictability
- Timing
- Fetal well-being
- Preservation of the pelvic floor (candidate should know, however, that caesarean section is not *totally* protective against urinary and bowel dysfunction later on).

8. ***Disadvantages of vaginal delivery*:** **10**

- Some women find labour distasteful
- May be an underlying psychosexual problem
- Pain
- Increased morbidity and mortality for fetus:
  — Intrapartum deaths — 2/1000
  — Asphyxial brain damage — 2/1000
  — Shoulder dystocia — 3/1000
- Pelvic floor/bladder/rectal trauma:
  — 20% women have new urinary symptoms for up to 12 months
  — 10% women have residual anal symptoms
  — ? incidence of prolapse

- May not deliver spontaneously:
  - 10% require emergency caesarean section
  - Emergency caesarean section 1.5 x more risky than elective CS
  - Up to 20% require instrumental vaginal delivery

Total mark out of 40: divide by 4 for final mark

STATION 7.8

Premature breech

Marks

Candidate's instructions

A 17-year-old patient is admitted in her first pregnancy at 28 weeks gestation. Her uterus is contracting every 3–4 minutes. On examination her cervix is 2–3 cm dilated and fully effaced with the membranes intact. An ultrasound scan is available which shows that the baby's size is appropriate for this gestation with a complete breech presentation. *What would your management be and how would you counsel the patient*?

Examiner's instructions

The candidate should make the diagnosis of premature labour with likely progress and delivery. He should be aware of the following:

- Survival at this gestation is 80% (with 10% serious morbidity), all else being equal.
- The value of administering steroids and delaying delivery until they have had a chance to have an effect.
- There is no evidence that caesarean section would benefit perinatal outcome.
- Caesarean section increases maternal morbidity and mortality.
- The risks of vaginal delivery with breech presentation — head entrapment by the cervix (rare but fatal).

The following should be assessed and marked:

1. **Immediate appraisal** — *What would you do in the first instance?*
   - Confirm clinical findings **1**
   - CTG to assess fetal condition (should understand shortcomings of such assessment in the premature fetus) **1**
   - Keep membranes intact **1**
   - Give steroids **1**
   - Tocolysis, to gain time for steroids to act. **1**

2. **Options for delivery** — *What are your clinical options, assuming assessment of mother and fetus do not indicate compromise?*

- Conservative management:
  - — Leave membranes intact **2**
  - — Tocolysis unlikely to delay delivery more than 72 hours **2**
  - — Time bought may be beneficial (*Why?*) **1**
- If labour progresses — vaginal delivery:
  - — Least risk to mother (short- and long-term) **1**
  - — Risk to fetus unpredictable **1**
  - — No clear evidence in literature of increased risk to the the fetus from vaginal delivery compared with caesarean section. **1**
  - — Recognized risk of cervical head entrapment **1**
  - — Maintaining membranes intact reduces risks **1**
- Caesarean section:
  - — Increased maternal morbidity and mortality **1**
  - — Risk increased for future pregnancy (consider maternal age), placenta praevia increased x 4 **1**
  - — Uncertain benefits for the fetus **1**
- Opinion on candidate's preferred option and why she chose it. **2**

3. **Counselling** — *How would you counsel the patient?* **10**

- Explain current situation
- High likelihood of progress towards delivery
- Survival at this gestation, all else being equal, is 80%+, with a 10% rate of serious handicap in those who survive
- Steroids reduce morbidity and mortality by up to 50%
- No clear-cut advantage for vaginal over caesarean delivery
- Vaginal delivery carries uncertainties for the baby
- Caesarean section carries uncertainties for the mother with potential risks for future pregnancies
- Seek mother's views and wishes.

Total mark out of 30: divide by 3 for final mark

STATION 7.9

Dilated fetal renal pelvis — role-play

Marks

Candidate's instructions

A routine ultrasound scan in one of your patients reveals a dilated fetal renal pelvis at 20 weeks gestation. You see your patient and her partner immediately after the scan. *How would you counsel them?*

Role-player's instructions

The mother should ask:

- *Is my baby normal?*
- *What happens now?*
- *What will happen after my baby is born?*

Examiner's instructions

Notes: Dilated renal pelvis may result from (presumed) intrauterine vesico–ureteric reflux or from the effects of maternal hormones on the fetal renal tract. A detailed ultrasound scan is necessary to exclude abnormalities of other systems. Repeat the ultrasound scan at 24, 28 and 34 weeks. Uncommonly, dilation will progress to involve the calyces. In a boy it is important to look at the fetal bladder wall — excess thickness suggests posterior urethral valves. Postnatally, if ultrasound findings persist, the baby will need an MCUG to exclude vesico–ureteric reflux (20% incidence if a first-degree relative is affected) and renogram to exclude partial obstruction to urinary flow. Prophylactic antibiotics are usually given to the baby postnatally to reduce the risk of urinary tract infection.

1. ***Examiner's assessment*:**

- Introduction **1**
- Puts patient at ease **1**
- Listens attentively **1**
- Explains condition **1**
- Uses plain English **1**
- Follows verbal and non-verbal clues **1**
- Explains intended actions **1**
- Appropriate eye contact **1**

2. ***Role-player's assessment*:**

- Confidence in candidate **1**
- 'I would like to see this doctor again'. **1**

Total mark out of 10

STATION 7.10

Cot death

Marks

Candidate's instructions

You have received the following letter:

> Dear Doctor,
>
> Booking Clinic Referral
>
> Please accept this lady for booking in her third pregnancy. She is now at 9 weeks, by LMP. She has a history of two cot deaths (at age 1 year and at 4 months) which occurred while she was living in Scotland. She has recently moved to our area.
>
> Yours sincerely,
>
> (GP)

Discuss with the examiner what factors you will consider at this consultation.

Examiner's instructions

The following should be explored and marks allocated as shown below:

- Obstetric history: previous pregnancies and deliveries; obstetric clinical risk factors; dating; plan for pregnancy management. **1**
- Family history: consanguinity; family history of neonatal or infant death or chronic disease. **1**
- Social history — stable partner? stable home? Any history of drug or alcohol abuse? **1**
- Medical diagnosis: 'cot death' is not a diagnosis but a loose term for unexplained death in infancy. **1**
- Cause of death may have been SIDS (sudden infant death syndrome), a condition related to cardiorespiratory instability of uncertain cause; an infection; trauma; an acute complication of a chronic condition; or an acute presentation of an inherited metabolic problem. There might also have been non-accidental injury leading to apparent SIDS. Full details (including PM findings) of the two babies must be obtained. **2**

- Risks for this baby: if previous diagnoses are unclear this child will require neonatal investigation and supervision. If the deaths *were* attributed to SIDS, the family will require support this time. They should be offered referral to the FSID (Foundation for the Study of Infant Deaths) which runs a health-visitor based 'care of next infant' (CONI) scheme — offers open access to clinical care plus monitoring by weighing or apnoea alarms as well as education in risk reduction (of smoking avoidance, nursery temperature and bedding advice, early attention to minor illness, benefits of breastfeeding). **2**
- Presentation and examiner discretion. **2**

Total mark out of 10

ORAL ASSESSMENT EXAMINATION

8

STATION 8.1

Operative complications at hysterectomy

Marks

Candidate's instructions

You are the gynaecology registrar performing what was considered to be a routine hysterectomy, with your SHO assisting. Your consultant, who was to assist you, has been called to the labour ward for an emergency but is confident of your ability to deal with the case and has asked you to proceed. The patient is a 45-year-old lady with severe dysmenorrhoea and menorrhagia. She is of normal build and has had no previous abdominal or pelvic surgery.

You have performed a routine Pfannenstiel incision and, much to your surprise, you find that she has marked endometriosis with the bladder adhering to the front of the uterus. The normal tissue planes in the broad ligament have been obliterated.

You proceed with caution but suspect that, in your attempts to deflect the bladder downwards, you have torn the bladder. The examiner will ask you questions on your management of this situation.

Examiner's instructions

This question presents the candidate with a scenario in which difficulties have arisen during what appeared (preoperatively) to be a straightforward hysterectomy, due to the presence of extensive endometriosis. A posterior bladder wall tear has resulted.

The candidate is asked to comment on the management in a logical, safe and effective manner; to offer an adequate explanation to the patient and relatives in lay terms postoperatively; and to describe the correct immediate and long-term management of such a case.

The following points should be discussed, and marks awarded as shown:

1. **Initial assessment:** *What would you do first?* **10**
   - Confirm suspected diagnosis (2 cm defect in posterior wall of bladder)
   - Contact consultant and/or urologist and await instructions
   - Consider subtotal hysterectomy.
2. **Acute management:** Your consultant has now arrived and asks, *How would you repair the bladder?* **10**

- Two-layer closure with an absorbable suture
- Appropriate antibiotics.

3. **Management of the tear:** It is decided that subtotal hysterectomy will be sufficient. *Describe your technique for completing this procedure.* **10**

   - Identify anatomy
   - Haemostasis
   - Cervical stump.

4. **Checks/closure:** Before finishing the operation, are there any other measures you would consider? **10**

   - Prevention of adhesions
   - Treatment of endometriosis
   - Check ovaries
   - ? Catheter
   - ? Drain.

5. ***How would you explain to the patient what happened during her operation?*** **10**

   - Would use appropriate language
   - Adhesions — endometriosis.

Total marks out of 50: divide by 5 for final mark

STATION 8.2

Urinary incontinence — role-play

Candidate's instructions

You have 15 minutes in which to obtain a history relevant to the patient's presenting complaint and discuss with the patient any investigations and treatment you feel will be necessary.

Role-player's instructions

You are 58 years old and have four children who were all born by vaginal delivery, the last one being a difficult rotational forceps delivery. The birth weights were 3.2 kg, 3.4 kg, 4.3 kg and 4.8 kg. Your youngest child is now 14 years old. Your periods stopped 8 years ago and you have not been using HRT. Over the past 4 years you have been troubled with urinary problems — you leak urine whenever you cough or sneeze.

Your daily fluid intake includes 7–8 cups of tea or coffee; you smoke 20/day; and you drink alcohol socially. You have no previous medical history.

You are fed up with the problem and want something done about it. A friend who had a similar problem has told you that when she went to the hospital the doctor told her to lose weight and stop smoking. You don't think these factors have anything to do with *your* incontinence.

Examiner's instructions

At this station the candidate will have 15 minutes in which to obtain a history relevant to the patient's presenting complaint. The candidate should also discuss any investigations and treatment they feel will be necessary with the patient. When the candidate has completed the history he may ask you for details of the physical examination and investigations, which you should provide as outlined below:

- General examination: obese, BMI 31
- Pelvic examination: poor muscle tone; no abnormality found
- Investigations:
  - — MSSU normal
  - — Urodynamic tests show genuine stress incontinence

The following should be discussed, and marked as shown:

1. ***History*** 5
   - Language (non-medical)
   - History of patient's main symptoms: duration, amount, associated factors, impact on lifestyle
   - Menses /menopause, HRT
   - Obstetric history
   - PMH, family and social histories.
2. ***Examination*** 5
   - General examination
   - Pelvic examination
   - Assessment of pelvic floor tone.
3. ***Investigations*** 5
   - MSU/ C&S
   - Fluid intake/output chart
   - Urodynamic investigations
   - Explanation of investigations.
4. ***Treatment*** 5
   - Weight loss
   - Smoking
   - Physiotherapy
   - Biofeedback
   - Drugs
   - Surgery
   - ?Nil (after discussion of options)
   - Explanation of treatment options.

Total mark out of 20: divide by 2 for final mark

STATION 8.3

Menorrhagia — role-play

Marks

Candidate's instructions

The patient you are about to see has been referred to your outpatient clinic by her GP. A copy of the referral letter is given below. Read the letter and obtain a relevant history from the patient. You should also discuss any investigations and treatment that you feel may be indicated.

The examiner will provide you with the results of the pelvic examination when requested.

> Dear Doctor,
>
> I would be grateful if you could see Mrs Flood (age 41). She has been having increasingly heavy periods over the last year and has failed to respond to medical therapy.
>
> Yours sincerely,
>
> (GP)

Role-player's instructions

You are 41 years old and have two children, both born by caesarean section because of fetal distress. Your periods have been getting heavier over the past year, since you were sterilized. You are happily married and work as a care assistant.

Your periods are regular, coming every 30 days but last up for to 8 days. The first 3 to 4 days are heavy, with clots and occasional soiling of your clothing. Staining of bed sheets is more frequent. For sanitary protection you need to use double maxi-pads most of the time. You experience some period pain which is usually mild and occurs during the period itself.

You find that your social activities are very restricted and you regularly take 1–2 days off work at the time of your period.

You developed a DVT while on the O/C pill 18 months ago. You were sterilized and had a normal smear taken one year ago.

Previous treatment: progestogens, Ponstan, Cyclokapron.

Examiner's instructions

At this station the candidate will have 15 minutes to obtain a history relevant to the patient's presenting complaint. When the candidate has completed the history he may ask you for details of a physical examination and you should tell the candidate that no abnormalities were found either on general examination or on pelvic examination. The following areas should be explored and marked as indicated:

1. ***History*** 5
   - Language (non-medical)
   - History of presenting symptoms
   - Sterilization
   - O/C pill and DVT
   - Medical treatment
   - Menses: cycle/duration, amount/protection, social/work, pain
   - Obstetric history
   - Family and social histories.
2. ***Investigations*** 5
   - Biopsy
   - Hysteroscopy
   - Full blood count
   - Vaginal scan
   - Thyroid function tests
   - Explanation of investigations.
3. ***Treatment*** 5
   - Ablation/resection — advantages and disadvantages
   - Levonorgestrel IUCD
   - Hysterectomy (? vaginal, ? abdominal)
   - Explanation of treatment options.

Role-player's marks. 5

Total mark out of 20: divide by 2 for final mark

STATION 8.4	
Combined oral contraceptive (COC) and epilepsy	Marks

Candidate's instructions

A patient suffering from idiopathic epilepsy which is well controlled on carbamazepine is referred to you for advice on contraception. Discuss with the examiner the advice you will give her.

Examiner's instructions

The following issues should be discussed, and marks allocated as shown:

- *General principle*: Drugs which are enzyme inducers (e.g. carbamazepine, phenobarbitone, phenytoin) lead to increased activity of specific enzyme systems. Other drugs (e.g. oestrogens and progestogens) metabolized by the same enzymes will therefore be eliminated more quickly and their therapeutic effects will be reduced. The blood concentration of the combined oral contraceptive pill (COC) and the progesterone only pill (POP) is reduced by up to 50% in women taking these drugs. **2**
- *COC*: The patient should be started on a preparation containing 50 μg of oestrogen. To ensure that ovulation has been inhibited, the serum progesterone concentration should be measured on day 21 of the first cycle on the COC (while the patient continues to use a barrier method). The progestogens in the pill do not interfere with this assay. If ovulation is not inhibited the dose should be increased to a dose containing 60 μg of oestrogen (two tablets of a 30 μg preparation) and, if necessary, to 80 μg (a 30 μg and a 50 μg tablet). **3**
- *POP*: The patient should take double the usual dose. **3**
- *Side-effects*: Because of the increased drug metabolism the incidence of side-effects with these higher doses is similar to that associated with the usual doses in other women. **3**
- The antiepileptic drug, sodium valproate is *not* an enzyme inducer and no alterations need to be made in O/C dosage in patients taking it. **2**
- *Depo-Provera*: Women on these parenteral progestogens are already on an adequate dose and do not require additional hormones. **3**

- *Progestogen-IUCDs*: These exert their effects locally and are not affected by antiepileptic drugs. 3
- *Barrier methods are* not affected by these drugs. 1

Total mark out of 20: divide by 2 for final mark

STATION 8.5

Factors predisposing to pre-eclampsia

Marks

Candidate's instructions

At this station you will discuss with the examiner the factors predisposing to pre-eclampsia (PET).

Examiner's instructions

Mark the discussion as follows:

- Primiparity 4
  - — Proteinuric PET occurs in 6% of first pregnancies and 2% of all second pregnancies
  - — Previous early miscarriage (or termination) does not offer protection
  - — Pregnancy by a new partner increases the risk to that of a first pregnancy.
- Previous obstetric history: If the first pregnancy was complicated with severe PET, the incidence in the second pregnancy rises to 12%. If, however, the first pregnancy was normotensive, the incidence is only 0.7% in the second pregnancy. 2
- Current obstetric history: Multiple pregnancy, hydatidiform mole and hydrops fetalis are associated with early (and severe) PET. 4
- Family history of PET: The risk is increased X2 if the patient's grandmother was affected, X3 if her sister was affected; and up to X4–5 if her mother was affected. 3
- Medical history: pre-existing hypertension, diabetes mellitus, autoimmune disorders, thrombophilias. 3
- Socio-economic factors: higher incidence with lower socio-economic class. 2
- Smoking: lower incidence in smokers, but if they *are* affected fetal outcome is poorer. 2

Total mark out of 20: divide by 2 for final mark

STATION 8.6

Counselling after caesarean section — role-play

Candidate's instructions

A 26-year-old patient is attending for a postnatal check-up. She had her first baby by emergency caesarean section six weeks ago. She has recovered normally and her baby is well. She is of normal stature and her baby weighed 3.65 kg at birth.

You are to provide new with her labour partogram which shows:

- Spontaneous labour
- Cephalic presentation — left occipitolateral
- Contractions 3:10
- Normal maternal and fetal observations
- Secondary arrest at 6 cm cervical dilatation
- Oxytocin used but no change over 3 hours
- FHR irregularities: CS performed.

She has some questions regarding her delivery. You are required to answer her queries and counsel her as you would do in your normal practice.

Role-player's instructions

Please ask the following questions:

- *Why did I need a caesarean delivery?*
- *What would have happened if I had not been delivered by caesarean?*
- *Why was I given a drip (oxytocin)?*
- *Will I need a caesarean section for future deliveries?*
- *Are there any tests which will tell me whether I can deliver vaginally in future?*
- *Are there any additional risks for future pregnancies as a result of this delivery?*

Examiner's instructions

These questions should be discussed, and your assessment of the interview marked as shown:

1. ***General assessment*** **5**
   - Language
   - Introduction
   - Eye contact and appropriate use of language
   - Listening and summarizing.
2. ***Why did I need a caesarean delivery?*** **5**
   - Progress in labour stopped
   - Possible causes: cephalopelvic disproportion or inefficient uterine activity; but often no apparent cause.
3. ***What would have happened if I had not been delivered by caesarean?*** **3**
   - Uterine inertia
   - Continued failure to make progress
   - Possible fetal and maternal distress in extreme cases.
4. ***Why was I given a drip (oxytocin)?*** **2**
   - To ensure that uterine activity was optimal.
5. ***Will I need a caesarean section for future deliveries?*** **5**
   - Two out of three women will deliver vaginally if allowed to labour in a future pregnancy
   - This has to be compared with over nine out of ten if vaginal delivery was achieved in the first delivery.
6. ***Are there any tests which will tell me whether I can deliver vaginally in future?*** **5**
   - X-ray pelvimetry has been shown to be of no value
   - Other forms of pelvimetry (CT scan and MRI) have yet to have proper evaluation.
7. ***Are there any additional risks for future pregnancies as a result of this delivery?*** **5**
   - Yes
   - Four-fold chance of placenta praevia
   - Increased risk of caesarean delivery next time
   - Just under 1% risk of scar complication if vaginal delivery attempted next time.

Total mark out of 30: divide by 3 for final mark

STATION 8.7	
Rhesus disease	Marks

Candidate's instructions

You see a lady at 12 weeks gestation in clinic. She has a history of one first trimester pregnancy loss. Booking bloods show her to be blood group A-negative with anti-D antibodies, 4 IU/ml. She and her partner ask what this test result will mean for her and her baby. Discuss this with the examiner.

Examiner's instructions

The following should be discussed, and marked as indicated:

	Marks
• The significant antibody level means that she has been immunized, possibly at the time of the previous pregnancy loss. (Was serology checked at the time? Did she receive anti-D?) A full medical history will elicit other possibilities, e.g. transfusion.	2
• IgG antibodies will affect the baby — causing red-cell haemolysis if the baby is Rhesus-positive. If her partner is homozygous (DD) this is inevitable; if he is heterozygous (dD) the baby may be Rhesus-negative and unaffected. The father's Rhesus genotype should be determined.	2
• Pregnancy monitoring will be by repeat serology and later ultrasound monitoring of fetal health. This should be done in a centre with expertise in the condition and her care may have to be transferred for this reason.	2
• Fetal interventions may include fetal blood sampling (to determine group), amniocentesis (to assess severity of fetal haemolysis by optical density assessment of amniotic fluid) and the possibility of either fetal transfusion or early delivery.	2
• If mildly affected, the baby will have early jaundice requiring phototherapy or possibly exchange transfusion with Rhesus-negative adult blood. If moderately affected, the baby may be anaemic and pale at delivery and require immediate exchange transfusion. In either case neonatal mortality is not significantly increased. If severely affected, however, the fetus may develop intrauterine anaemia and hydrops — this risk can be minimized by monitoring the pregnancy and by fetal transfusion.	2
Total mark out of 10	

STATION 8.8

GnRH agonists

Marks

Candidate's instructions

Discuss the use of gonadotrophin-releasing hormone agonists in gynaecology with the examiner.

Examiner's instructions

The following should be discussed and marks allocated as shown below:

- GnRH-agonists are synthesized by substituting certain amino acids in the original decapeptide GnRH. They lead to an initial flare-up effect, increasing both gonadotrophins and oestrogen production for a few days. This is followed by a hypogonadotrophic hypo-oestrogenic state. 2
- Used in *endometriosis*: for symptomatic relief; postoperatively, to reduce (or delay) recurrence; preoperatively in extensive cases to make surgery technically easier. No improvement in fertility. 2
- Used in the management of *fibroids* — about 50% shrinkage in size, and reduction of menstrual loss. Used preoperatively to make surgery technically easier. 2
- Used in intractable cases of *premenstrual syndrome*. 2
- Used with gonadotrophins for the *induction of ovulation/superovulation*. There are three protocols: 8

  — *Long*: started during the previous cycle. Down-regulation is achieved before starting the gonadotrophin administration. *Advantages*: prevention of premature LH surge, control of cycle (for scheduling of egg collection in IVF).

  Disadvantages: requires higher doses of gonadotrophins and there is probably a higher incidence of ovarian hyperstimulation syndrome.

  — *Short*: started at the beginning of the cycle (day 1) followed by gonadotrophins (day 2 or 3).

  Advantages: prevention of premature LH surge (but not as good as with long protocol); requires lower doses of gonadotrophins (makes use of the flare-up effect).

  Disadvantages: probably has lower success rate in IVF compared with the long protocol.

— Ultra-short: started at the beginning of the cycle and given for a few days only.

Advantages: requires lower doses of gonadotrophins (makes use of the flare-up effect).

Disadvantages: no prevention of premature LH surge; more difficult scheduling.

- *Side-effects:* menopausal-like symptoms (hot flushes, night sweats, irritability, mood swings), osteoporosis if used over a prolonged period (> 24 weeks). 2
- *Role of add-back therapy:* reduces side-effects without affecting efficacy in endometriosis and PMS. 2

STATION 8.9

Elective caesarean section at 37 weeks

Marks

Candidate's instructions

Your patient, who is presently at 34 weeks gestation in an uncomplicated pregnancy, asks if she can have her planned (elective) caesarean section at 37+0 weeks instead of at 39 weeks as she hopes to attend an important business conference the following week. The caesarean section is being performed because of maternal request. She was fully counselled on elective caesarean section and the decision made some time ago. Discuss with the examiner the points you would cover in deciding the *timing* of the operation.

Examiner's instructions

The following points should be discussed, and marked as shown:

- At first sight there is no reason why this lady should not attend the conference while 38 weeks pregnant unless this involves an air flight. Details regarding this option and the importance of the engagement should be explored. **2**
- Hazards to the mother of planned operative delivery are little different at the two gestations. **1**
- The risks of requiring neonatal unit admission due to respiratory morbidity rise from 1.8% for planned caesarean section at 39 weeks to 4.2% at 38 weeks and 7.3% at 37 weeks. **2**
- The baby may develop respiratory distress syndrome which itself may be complicated (10% air leak; possible need for CPAP or IPPV). Jaundice may require phototherapy, delaying neonatal discharge. Poor feeding may necessitate the use of tube feeds and decrease the chance of successful establishment of breastfeeding. There is no guarantee that the baby will be fit for discharge in one week. **2**
- Your patient's request should be discouraged unless circumstances are exceptional. **2**
- Presentation and examiner's discretion. **1**

Total mark out of 10

STATION 8.10

Preterm labour

Marks

Candidate's instructions

A primigravid 25-year-old woman presents in established labour at 23 weeks + 5 days gestation with a cephalic presentation. You are asked to go and counsel her. Discuss with the examiner the key points you will cover.

Examiner's instructions

The following should be discussed and marks allocated as indicated:

- At 23 weeks, this baby would have a 50% chance of survival to admission for neonatal intensive care and an overall 12% chance of survival to discharge. At 24 weeks, equivalent figures would be 82% and 26%. (UK figures, EPICURE study). It is important to know the current figures for your own institution. **2**
- There is no evidence that delivery by caesarean section is of benefit in these circumstances. **2**
- The baby's chances are optimized by delivery in a centre with facilities for long-term neonatal intensive care — this should be arranged and availability of a cot confirmed. **2**
- Increased maturation is the most important factor affecting survival. **2**
- Steroids will enhance the chance of a liveborn baby's survival and ritodrine (or equivalent) should be given in an attempt to delay delivery until at least 24 hours after steroid administration — or for longer if possible, unless there is clinical evidence of maternal infection. **2**
- The neurodevelopmental outcome at this gestation is a significant consideration: 50% of survivors will have no disability; 25% mild disability; 25% serere disability. Problems may be multiple and affect development, neuromotor ability, vision or hearing. **2**
- Paediatricians should be alerted to come and counsel the couple so that they are fully aware of these figures. **2**

- Once the baby is born, other factors will influence the chance of intact survival — sex of the child, severity of lung disease, development of intracranial lesions, development of retinopathy and ethnicity. The ethos of the institution and parental wishes will influence the decision about when intensive care may be discontinued in the face of a predicted poor outcome. 2
- Presentation and examiner's discretion. 4

Total mark out of 20: divide by 2 for final mark

ORAL ASSESSMENT EXAMINATION

9

STATION 9.1

Macrosomia and shoulder dystocia

Marks

Candidate's instructions

You have been asked to see a patient whose symphysial–fundal height is above the 97th centile for gestational age at 40 weeks gestation. She has had two uncomplicated pregnancies in the past. In both she delivered vaginally 5–7 days after her expected date of delivery. Her first baby, female, weighed 3.8 kg (8 lbs 7 oz) and her second, female, 4.26 kg (9 lbs 6 oz). She is now at her expected date of delivery. There is a cephalic presentation with head three-fifths palpable.

Discuss the options for her management.

Examiner's instructions

The candidate should be aware of:

- The factors associated with shoulder dystocia:
  - — Macrosomia
  - — Multiparity
  - — Postmaturity
- The increased morbidity of shoulder dystocia
- The vagaries of weight estimation by ultrasound
- The unreliability of cervicography to predict shoulder dystocia.

Marks should be awarded as shown below for answers to the following questions:

1. ***What are the risk factors in this case?*** *5*

- Likelihood of macrosomia — observation of large-for-dates
- Multiparity — tendency for birthweight to rise with parity
- Big female babies in the past: males larger than females and this fetus could be male; post-date could lead to even higher birthweight.

2. ***What would you do next from the clinical standpoint?*** *5*

- Confirm clinical findings
- Associated features:

— maternal stature

— Check for possible glucose intolerance

- *Is it possible to estimate the birthweight?*

— Clinical estimation

— Ultrasound: 15% error, less reliable indicator with large fetuses; only 2–4% chance of shoulder dystocia if > 4 kg; not a good predictor.

3. ***What are your management options?*** **5**

- Await spontaneous labour: the fetus continues to grow but spontaneous labour offers the best chance of vaginal delivery
- Induction of labour: this prevents further increment in size but introduces the uncertainties of induction
- Caesarean section: reduces risk of shoulder dystocia but increases maternal morbidity and mortality, and there is still increased risk of neonatal morbidity
- None of these options have been shown to be superior to any of the others.

4. ***What would you do in anticipation of a vaginal delivery?*** **5**

- Plan the labour management
- Remember and warn staff that normal cervimetric progress does not exclude shoulder dystocia
- Look out for delay in progress either in first or second stages
- Ensure clear communication with delivery suite team
- Prepare contingency plan should shoulder dystocia occur: trained and experienced staff should be available at delivery.

Total mark out of 20: divide by 2 for final mark

STATION 9.2

Postoperative patient counselling — preparatory station

Candidate's instructions

You are the consultant in charge and have just returned from your holiday. You find the following letter on your desk:

> Dear Colleague,
>
> Re. Amanda Barton (d.o.b. 22/7/74)
>
> This patient came to see me today in considerable distress. She tells me that she attended A&E, late at night, 2 weeks ago with severe pain. I gather that she was admitted to the Gynaecology Unit, but neither reviewed nor offered analgesia until the following morning. She then apparently collapsed and underwent emergency surgery for what she was told was 'a problem pregnancy.' She was discharged two days later without adequate explanation and told to make an appointment to see us to have the stitches removed. I have received no information about this episode whatsoever.
>
> May I request that you see this patient at your earliest convenience to discuss her care and furnish me with a suitable discharge summary.
>
> Yours sincerely,
>
> (GP)

Your secretary has arranged for the patient to see you today. You have not been able to speak to Dr Jones (on leave) or Mr Phillips (on nights). Prepare to counsel the patient at the next station.

Entries in the hospital notes read as follows:

PATIENT NOTES

11/5/2000 **23.41** 26-year-old female, c/o abdo. pain for 6 hours
Pain getting worse and exacerbated by movement
Vomited x1
O/E: maximal tenderness RIF, rebound+, no guarding
P 90, BP 110/70, T 37.2°
DD: appendix, UTI, ectopic
Inv. — urine analysis
— preg. test
— FBC, G&S

Dr Smith, SHO, A&E

12/5/2000	**00.18**	Urine: NAD Preg.test. POSITIVE FBC: Hb 124, WCC 8.3, Plt 291 D/w Dr Jones (O&G Reg) — busy in theatre at present, advised admit to Gynae Unit for review *Dr Smith, SHO, A&E*
12/5/00	**01.25**	Patient received on Ward 8 ? Ectopic pregnancy P 95, BP 110/70 C/o abdo. pain Drs asked to review *E. Green, RGN*
12/5/00	**01.55**	Still c/o pain Drs called again Drs in theatre for C/S — verbal message to give co-dydramol 2 co-dydramol given as instructed *E.Green, RGN*
Day shift		
12/5/00	**07.35**	P 95, BP 110/65, T 36.8° C/o worsening abdo. pain No analgesia prescribed Keep NBM and await medical review *T. Hunter, RGN*
12/5/00	**08.45**	WR, Mr Phillips (Reg) Hx as above (+ve UPT, LMP 7 weeks, abdo. pain, no bleeding) Obs stable P/A – Tender lower abdo. with rebound and slight guarding Spec. — NAD, triple swabs taken P/V — small A/V uterus, cx excitation ++, no masses *Imp*. Possible ectopic *Plan*: analgesia, U/S and review with result *Dr Lamour, SHO*
12/5/00	**09.05**	Pethidine given as prescribed *T. Hunter, RGN*
12/5/00	**13.05**	Crash-bleeped to U/S dept. approx. 11.25 Pt collapsed, pale, sweaty. P 110, BP 90/40 U/S incomplete, but uterus empty on T/A scan: likely ruptured ectopic IVI sited by anaesthetist, FBS and G&S sent, 2 unit X-match req. Pt transferred to theatre *Phillips, Reg* *Written in retrospect*

12/5/00	**14.05**	Received onto Ward 8 from Recovery P 75, BP 110/65, T 36.2°. Comfortable *Flint, RGN*
13/5/00	**08.34**	Comfortable postop. BS present *Plan*: IVI down, cath. out, eat and drink, mobilize *Ali, SHO*
14/5/00	**08.51**	Day 2, eating and drinking, mobile *Plan*: home p.m., GP to take stitches out *Lamour, SHO*

THEATRE NOTES

Surgeons:	Phillips / Lamour
Anaesthetist:	Lasakin
Indication:	Suspected ruptured ectopic
Findings:	600 ml haemoperitoneum
	Ruptured R. tubal ectopic
Procedure:	GA
	Swab, drape, cath.
	Routine laparoscopy through subumbilical incision — blood +++
	Converted to laparotomy:
	Modified Cohen's incision
	R salpingectomy
	Abdomen washed out with warm saline
	Routine closure
	All ties and sutures — Vicryl. Skin — clips
	Foley catheter inserted
Post Op:	Fluids as per anaesth.
	Catheter 1/7
	Clips 5/7

Phillips, Reg.

DRUG CHART

Once Only:

11/5/00	01.55	Co-dydramol 2	*E. Green*
12/5/00	15.30	'Anti-D 250 iu	*I. Hunter*

PRN:

Pethidine	50 mg	09.05	12/5/00	*I. Hunter*
Stemetil	12.5 mg	09.05	12/5/00	*I. Hunter*
	12.5 mg	22.10	12/5/00	*J. Oliver*
	12.5 mg	06.20	13/5/00	*J. Oliver*
Morphine	10 mg	16.00	12/5/00	*I. Hunter*
	10 mg	22.10	12/5/00	*J. Oliver*
	10 mg	06.20	13/5/00	*J. Oliver*
Voltarol	50 mg	09.05	13/5/00	*I. Hunter*
	50 mg	17.20	13/5/00	*I. Hunter*
	50 mg	07.30	14/5/00	*M. Cox*
	50 mg	15.30	14/5/00	*M. Cox*
Co-dydramol	2 tabs	12.45	13.5.00	*I. Hunter*
	2 tabs	21.20	13/5/00	*J. Oliver*
	2 tabs	12.30	14/5/00	*M. Cox*

FLUID CHART

12/5/00	N. Saline	1000 ml	*In theatre*
12/5/00	Gelfusin	500 ml	*In theatre*
12/5/00	Gelfusin	500 ml	*In theatre*
12/5/00	Hartmann's	1000 ml	*In theatre*
12/5/00	Hartmann's	1000 ml	8-hourly (13.51–19.35)
12/5/00	N. Saline	1000 ml	8-hourly (19.45–08.20)

RESULTS

	FBC	Hb (g/L)	WCC ($x10^9$/l)	Platelets ($x10^9$/l)
12/5/00	00.15	124	8.3	291
12/5/00	11.55	103	10.4	329

Blood Group: A Rh-positive

STATION 9.3

Postoperative patient counselling — examination station

Candidate's instructions

Counsel the patient whose details were presented at the previous station.

Examiner's instructions

The following should be discussed and marks allocated as shown:

	Marks
1. ***Explanation to the patient*:**	
• Reason for admission (suspected ectopic pregnancy)	1
• Reason for delay in gynaecology review (in theatre, not re-bleeped later)	1
• Reason for U/S (to exclude viable pregnancy)	1
• Reason for collapse (the ectopic ruptured)	1
• Reason for operation (to stop internal bleeding)	1
• Operation (laparoscopy had to be abandoned; right tube removed).	1
2. ***Apology*:**	
• Delay in gynaecology review (*action* — will speak to nursing and medical staff involved)	1
• Delay in adequate analgesia (*action* — will speak to nursing and medical staff)	1
• Apparent lack of information postoperatively and on discharge (*action* — will discuss with nursing and medical staff; will review ward policy if necessary)	1
• Lack of personal involvement (on leave — seen at first possible opportunity).	1
3. ***Issues*:**	
• Ability to listen to patient and respond appropriately	2
• Laparoscopy *vs.* laparotomy	1
• Causes of ectopic (need to chase swab results)	1
• Future fertility (offer early HSG, scan)	1

- Check Hb (patient will complain of tiredness) **1**
- Check blood group and discuss with haematologist (Rh +ve / anti-D given) **1**
- Contraception **1**
- Promise to write to the GP **1**
- Offer further follow-up. **1**

Up to 5 marks may be *deducted* for any inappropriate criticism of other members of staff — the consultant (candidate) has not spoken to them yet.

Total mark out of 20: divide by 2 for final mark

STATION 9.4

Results and histories — preparatory station

Candidate's instructions

You are a specialist registrar (SpR 2) and your consultant is away. The secretary gives you the following results and histories. There are 10 altogether. Prepare to discuss the diagnosis and further management in each case with the examiner at the next station.

1. A 47-year-old lady who presented with secondary amenorrhoea. Clinically she was noted to be hirsute and a blood pressure of 160/110 mmHg had been recorded.

   Testosterone: 20 nmol/l.

2. A couple with a history of three consecutive miscarriages. The female partner is known to carry a balanced (Robertsonian) translocation.

   Report from CVS carried out at 14 weeks in current pregnancy: 46 XY (7q+, 14q−). This is a male karyotype showing the same balanced translocation seen in the maternal karyotype.

3. Clinical history: ERPC approx. 8 weeks, incomplete miscarriage.

   Histology report: Stella-Arias reaction. No chorionic villi seen.

4. Booking results for a patient at 14 weeks gestation with a history of unexplained previous mid-trimester pregnancy loss.

   MSU: RBC < 10; WBC 30/ml; heavy growth of group F *Streptococcus*.

5. *Cervical cytology report*: 'Unsatisfactory smear — suggest repeat in six months'.

6. A 45-year-old patient who presented with menorrhagia. A family history of breast carcinoma was noted.

   FBC results:

   Hb — 105 g/l
   WBC — 6.5×10^9/l
   Platelets — 415×10^9/l
   RBC — 4.29×10^{12}/l
   HCT — 39.7%
   MCV — 92.5 fl
   MCH — 32.0 pg
   MCHC — 346 g/l
   RDW — 13.7%
   MPV — 8.7 fl

7. Booking results from a G2 P1 patient at 14 weeks gestation. The patient has a history of receiving a blood transfusion following a road traffic accident.

   Blood Group: A Rh-negative.

   Antibodies: c — 2 iu/l.

8. Results from investigations into primary infertility.

   Semen analysis:

   Volume — 3.5 ml

   Ph — 7.3

   Sperm concentration — 32 x 10^6/ml

   Motility — 63% forward progression

   Morphology — 35% abnormal forms.

   Day 21 Progesterone: 11 nmol/l.

9. A 61-year-old patient presenting with a pelvic mass.

   CA125: 1500 u/l.

10. A 24-year-old G1 P0 at 26 weeks gestation.

    Glucose tolerance test report (75 g load)

    (Indication: family history)

    Fasting — 6.2 mmol/l

    1 Hour — 10.8 mmol/l

    2 Hours — 8.5 mmol/l

STATION 9.5	
Results and histories — examination station	Marks

Examiner's instructions

With reference to the information received at the previous station, the following points should be discussed about each report, and marked as shown:

1. ***Secondary amenorrhoea*:**
   - History of sudden-onset hirsutism, secondary amenorrhoea, hypertension and elevated testosterone suggests either an ovarian or an adrenal tumour. **1**
   - Advice from the oncologists should be sought without delay. **1**
   - Urgent MRI of ovaries and adrenal should be arranged (MRI best, CT and ultrasound are alternatives). **1**
2. ***Genetic counselling after previous repeated miscarriage*:**
   - Balanced translocation passed from mother to fetus. Since mother is normal this should have no implications for the development of the fetus. **2**
   - The candidate should ensure that the couple are notified of the result and reassured appropriately. **1**
3. ***Histology report after ERCP***
   - History of ERPC at 8 weeks for incomplete miscarriage. Histology suggests an ectopic pregnancy. **1**
   - The candidate should arrange immediate (same day) review of the patient with a quantitative serum HCG and transvaginal U/S. **2**
4. ***MSU in patient with previous unexplained mid-trimester pregnancy loss*:**
   - Probably asymptomatic UTI at 14 weeks with a history of mid-trimester loss. **1**
   - Asymptomatic UTIs are associated with pregnancy loss — the candidate should contact the patient and arrange for treatment (non-urgent, could write). **2**
5. ***Unsatisfactory smear report*:**
   - Unsatisfactory smear report — candidate needs to request patient's notes. **1**

- If there has been clinical suspicion of a lesion, colposcopy may be appropriate — otherwise repeat in six months as advised. **2**

6. ***Family history of breast cancer in a patient with menorrhagia, FBC report*:**
   - Normocytic anaemia in a woman with menorrhagia and a family history of breast cancer. **1**
   - Breast cancer needs to be excluded as a cause for the anaemia. **1**
   - Clinical breast examination should be performed (if not done already) and the family history documented. Specialist advice should be sought. **1**

7. ***Booking blood results*:**
   - Anti-c antibodies in a Rh-negative parous patient with a history of blood transfusion. The antibodies could have come either from iso-immunization or from the blood transfusion. **1**
   - Anti-c can cause immune hydrops and the report needs to be acted upon. The father's blood group should be checked and advice sought from the regional Rhesus clinic. Maternal antibodies should be rechecked in 2 weeks. Rising titres warrant referral to the regional centre. **2**

8. ***Primary infertility investigation results*:**
   - Infertile couple with normal semen analysis, and a low day-21 progesterone level suggesting anovulation. **1**
   - Need FSH, LH, testosterone, prolactin and TSH levels and ovarian ultrasound to investigate the cause. Non-urgent review. **2**

9. ***CA125 results in patient with a pelvic mass*:**
   - Pelvic mass in a 61-year-old with an elevated CA125: diagnosis is ovarian cancer until proven otherwise. **1**
   - Arrange urgent pelvic U/S and liaise with gynae-oncologists. **2**

10. ***Glucose tolerance test results*:**
    - Impaired glucose tolerance at 26 weeks gestation. **1**
    - Needs urgent referral to joint diabetic clinic for advice (about diet) and monitoring (BM stix, glycosylated Hb, random blood sugars, fetal U/S biometry). May need insulin. **2**

Total mark out of 30: divide by 3 for final mark

STATION 9.6

Urinary incontinence

Marks

Candidate's instructions

A 45-year-old woman presents with an 8-year history of stress incontinence with some urgency and, very occasionally, urge incontinence. She has had physiotherapy without much success.

What investigations would you order? On the basis of the investigation results you will be provided with, how would you manage this patient?

Examiner's instructions

The following points should be discussed, and marked as shown:

1. ***Investigations required*:** **6**
   - MSU/nitrite dipstick
   - Frequency volume chart
   - Urodynamics.

   The candidate is then given the following report:

   Urodynamics show an initial void of 150 ml with a peak flow of 12 ml/sec. There is a prolonged voiding curve with three separate voids. There is a residual volume of 110 ml. Her bladder is stable and she tolerates 300 ml. Provocation demonstrates severe genuine stress incontinence. At the end she voids with a pressure of 15 cm H_2O and again has an interrupted stream, with a peak flow of 11 ml/sec and a residual volume of 95 ml.

2. ***Comments on the investigation results*:** **6**
   - UDA shows GSI.
   - The free-flow rate suggests a poor flow rate which may be due to a failing detrusor. This is a risk factor for voiding difficulties if the patient was to be operated on.
   - She shows mixed symptoms and the reduced capacity of 300 ml may be important. This may be part of the pathology or secondary to her repeated emptying, which she does to avoid leaking.

3. ***Management options***: 6

   - Given the risk of voiding difficulties this woman should be taught clean intermittent self-catheterization prior to any surgery.
   - She may be a good candidate for a conservative device such as a plug or a tampon, which would avoid the risk of retention.
   - The other reason to avoid surgery is the worrying irritative symptoms and a reduced bladder capacity.
   - At least, she needs to be counselled that these symptoms may worsen after surgery.
   - Treatment of the irritative symptoms with an anticholinergic medication could precipitate voiding dysfunction because of the potentially failing detrusor.
   - However, bladder drill may be appropriate as this does not carry a risk of voiding difficulties. This could be done in conjunction with a pelvic-floor assessment to try and establish whether the previous exercises were effective.

4. ***Further investigations*** with either ambulatory urodynamics or bladder wall thickness measurement may be indicated or a pad test to assess how much leakage occurs. 2

Total mark out of 20: divide by 2 for final mark

STATION 9.7

Induction of ovulation

Marks

Candidate's instructions

Discuss with the examiner the methods that would be used for induction of ovulation in an anovulatory woman with polycystic ovarian disease.

Examiner's instructions

The following should be discussed and marks allocated as indicated:

1. ***Clomifene*:** **9**
   - Dosage (50–150 mg/day) and how it is used (orally for 5 days, beginning on day 2,3,4 or 5 of the cycle)
   - Side-effects (oestrogenic and anti-oestrogenic, OHSS)
   - Results (approx. 70% will ovulate and approx. 40% will conceive, over a 6-month treatment period)
   - Monitoring (the establishment of regular menstrual cycles/ mid-luteal progesterone)
   - Risk of multiple pregnancy (8–10%).
2. ***Gonadotrophins*:** **9**
   - Dosage (50–75 IU/day) and how it is used (SC or IM depending on the preparation used, starting day 2 of the cycle)
   - Side-effects (OHSS)
   - Results (approx. 90% will ovulate and approx. 40% will conceive, over a 6-month treatment period)
   - Monitoring (oestradiol measurement and ovarian U/S)
   - Risk of multiple pregnancy (10–20%).
3. ***Laparoscopic ovarian drilling*:** **9**
   - Number of drills in each ovary, duration, and diathermy setting. One method is 4 drills, each for 4 seconds at 40 watts
   - Side-effects (5–15% peri-ovarian adhesions and complications of laparoscopy)
   - Results (approx. 70% will ovulate spontaneously and the remaining will be more responsive to clomifene. Over half of those who ovulate will conceive)

- Monitoring (the establishment of regular menstrual cycles/mid-luteal progesterone)
- Risk of multiple pregnancy due to treatment is nil.

4. ***Metformin.*** 3

Total mark out of 30: divide by 3 for final mark

STATION 9.8

Fetal abnormality — role-play

Candidate's instructions

You are the obstetric consultant in the antenatal clinic. You are asked to see a patient who has just returned from the ultrasound department, where her routine 20-week scan has been performed.

The scan shows an abnormal fetus and the report is shown below:

Ultrasound Report: Karen Smith

Menstrual dates: 20 weeks

BPD: 42 mm

Femur length: 29 mm

Abdominal circumference: 125 mm

Fetal heart beat: present

There are bilateral choroid plexus cysts measuring >1 cm. In addition, there is a small omphalocele and the hands appear clenched with overlapping digits.

A quick review of the notes indicates that Karen Smith is a healthy, 23-year-old primigravida, with no previous medical or surgical history and no family history of congenital abnormalities. She booked early with the GP and attended the hospital antenatal clinic at 15 weeks (your usual practice). She declined Down's syndrome screening as a friend had miscarried a normal fetus following an amniocentesis after a positive screening test.

Explain the scan findings to Mrs Smith and discuss with her how the pregnancy might be managed from now on. You will be awarded marks for your ability to communicate with Mrs Smith and for giving appropriate advice.

Role-player's instructions

You are Karen Smith, a 23-year-old shop worker. You married 2 years ago and used sheath contraception until 9 months ago, when you started trying for a baby.

Your periods are regular, last 5 days and occur every 28 days. Your last period was on 10/6/98, of which you are certain, and the baby is due on 17/3/99.

You went to the GP when your period was 2 weeks late and had a positive pregnancy test. The GP took pulse and blood pressure, (both normal), weighed you (60 kg 9 stone 5 lb), and measured your height (1.65 m — 5′ , 5″).

You had a further visit to the GP at 12 weeks and met the midwife. Again the results of your examination were normal and you were told that the womb could just be felt in your abdomen.

At 15 weeks you went to the hospital clinic for the first time and were told that everything was normal. You had a number of blood tests, but declined the Down's syndrome screening test as a friend from work had had the test which was positive and had an amnio., but lost the baby a few days later. The baby turned out to be normal. You have no confidence in the screening test and do not want to risk losing your baby.

You had a scan earlier today and have come to the clinic to discuss the result with the consultant. You do not at this point suspect that there is anything wrong.

You should not initiate conversation with the candidate.

Examiner's instructions

The following should be assessed and marks allocated as shown below:

1. ***Communication skills***: **10**
   - Appropriate introduction
   - Sympathetic approach
   - Encouraging the patient to ask questions
   - Listening
   - Avoidance of medical jargon.

2. ***Advice/comments***: **10**
   - Correct description of abnormalities
   - Mid-trimester IUGR
   - Suggestive of chromosomal abnormality (trisomy 18)
   - Offer second consultation with husband present
   - Offer counselling
   - Offer amnio.
   - Emphasize relative risks of abnormality *vs* amnio.

- Choroid plexus cysts + two other abnormalities carries >10% risk trisomy 18.

Total mark out of 20: divide by 2 for final mark

STATION 9.9

Upper segment caesarean section

Marks

Candidate's instructions

Discuss with the examiner the indications for upper segment caesarean section in modern obstetrics.

Examiner's instructions

The following should be discussed and marks allocated as shown:

	Marks
• Peri-/post-mortem CS	2
• Extreme prematurity (no well-formed lower segment)	2
• Caesarean Wertheim hysterectomy (for Ca cervix)	2
• Inaccessible lower segment (e.g. fibroids, extensive adhesions)	2
• Impacted fetal shoulder.	2

Total mark out of 10

STATION 9.10

Maternal mortality: definitions

Marks

Candidate's instructions

Discuss with the examiner the definitions of the following terms: maternal death, direct maternal death, indirect maternal death, late maternal death, fortuitous maternal death, and maternal mortality rate.

Examiner's instructions

- *Maternal death*: the death of a woman while pregnant or within 42 days of delivery or abortion, irrespective of the duration or site of pregnancy, from any cause related to or aggravated by the pregnancy or its management (excluding accidental or incidental causes). **2**
- *Direct death*: death resulting from obstetric complications of pregnancy, labour or the puerperium; from interventions, omissions, incorrect treatment, or from a chain of events resulting from any of these. **2**
- *Indirect death*: death resulting from pre-existing disease, or a condition arising during pregnancy not due to direct obstetric cause but aggravated by the physiological changes that occur in pregnancy. **2**
- *Late maternal death*: death occurring between 42 days and 1 year after abortion or delivery, due to direct or indirect causes. **1**
- *Fortuitous maternal death*: death due to causes unrelated to (but occurring in) pregnancy, labour or the puerperium. **1**
- *Maternal mortality rate*: the number of maternal deaths per million 'maternities' (i.e. pregnancies, whether resulting in childbirth or abortion). **2**

Total mark out of 10

ORAL ASSESSMENT EXAMINATION

10

STATION 10.1	
Breastfeeding	Marks

Candidate's instructions

You are asked to suggest ways of increasing the rate of successful breastfeeding in mothers delivering at your hospital. *What would you consider to be important aspects of hospital and community policies on breastfeeding?*

Examiner's instructions

Background information:

- Over 60% of UK women initiate breastfeeding at birth but this declines rapidly within the first 3 weeks.
- 25% of women who wish to breastfeed fail to do so.
- Conflicting advice and lack of support by health professionals are stated by women as relevant factors in breastfeeding difficulties and failure.

The candidate should be aware of the WHO/UNICEF '10 steps to successful breastfeeding' recommendations which provide a model for organizations to use:

- Have a written breastfeeding policy of which all health care staff are aware. 1
- Train staff in the skills required to implement the policy. 1
- Inform all pregnant women about the benefits to mother and baby and the management of breastfeeding: benefits to the baby include protection against some allergies and some infections, and possible decreased infant mortality; benefits to the mother include reduced ovarian and breast cancer risks, and pregnancy spacing. 1
- Help mothers initiate breastfeeding within 30 minutes of birth. 1
- Show mothers how to breastfeed and how to maintain lactation (by expression) if they are separated from the baby. 1
- Babies should not be given any other food or drink unless medically indicated. 1
- Keep mothers and babies together 24 hours a day while in hospital. 1

- Encourage breastfeeding on demand. 1
- Avoid pacifiers (dummies) in newborn breastfeeding infants. 1
- Know about breastfeeding support groups and inform mothers about them. 1

Total mark out of 10

STATION 10.2	
Speculum examination	Marks

Candidate's instructions

You are provided with two vaginal specula, a Cusco's and a Sims'. Discuss their use with the examiner.

Examiner's instructions

The following points should be discussed:

- Speculum examination allows inspection of the vaginal walls and the cervix. 3
- *Traditionally, this inspection is carried out before palpation (bimanual examination).* The advantage of this sequence of examination is that lesions of the cervix and the vagina will be undisturbed before being inspected. Some lesions can bleed on touch making subsequent inspection unsatisfactory and cervical cytological examination inadequate. On the other hand, some gynaecologists perform a gentle bimanual examination first to assess the size of the vagina in order to choose the appropriate size of the speculum. 3
- The size of speculum required can be judged fairly accurately from the patient's history of coitus, the use of tampons, pregnancies, deliveries and prolapse. Inspection of the introitus will also give an indication of the size of the vagina. 3
- The Cusco's is self-retaining, so that both hands are free for other tasks, but it does not allow adequate inspection of the vaginal walls — particularly the anterior and posterior. 3
- The Sims' allows direct inspection of the anterior and lateral vaginal walls and, as it is being withdrawn, the posterior vaginal wall comes into view. Sims' speculum examination is, therefore, essential in cases of prolapse, incontinence or suspected vaginal fistula. 3
- Before inserting the speculum in the vagina you should warm it by squeezing it in your gloved hands for a few seconds, and then apply a thin layer of non-greasy lubricant to its outer surface. 3
- The Cusco's speculum is used with the patient in the dorsal position, and the Sim's speculum in the Sims' or left-lateral position. 3

- A common error is to insert the speculum obliquely or longitudinally in line with the vulval cleft, and then rotate it in the vagina. This can cause painful pressure on the urethra and should be avoided. The correct method of application is to separate the labia minora with the fingers of one hand and insert the speculum *directly* (blades transverse) with the other. This is because the vagina is wider from side to side. While inserting the speculum you should keep an eye on the patient's face to detect any pain or discomfort you might be causing her. 3

- With the Cusco's speculum it is a matter of personal choice whether you insert it with the handles pointing upwards or downwards — each has its merits. If the handles are pointing downwards they will fit snugly into the anal cleft and the speculum can be inserted more deeply than it can if the handles point upwards (when they will be checked by the symphysis pubis). However, if the patient is in the dorsal position on a soft-mattress bed it is likely that her buttocks will sink into the mattress, which will hinder the insertion of the speculum if its handles are pointing downwards. 3

- After inserting the speculum you would observe the state of the vaginal walls and the cervix. You would ask the patient to cough a few times and note any abnormal bulging of the vaginal walls or descent of the cervix. You should also be looking out for the presence of any ulceration, swelling, discharge, bleeding, cervical ectopy or the threads of an intrauterine contraceptive device. 3

Total mark out of 30: divide by 3 for final mark

STATION 10.3	
Positions for pelvic examination	Marks

Candidate's instructions

Discuss with the examiner what patient positions are used for pelvic examination in the outpatient clinic.

Examiner's instruction

These three positions should be described, and the discussion marked as shown:

1. The ***dorsal position*** is the one most commonly used. In this position the patient is lying on her back, her hips are flexed and abducted, and the knees flexed. This position allows adequate inspection of the vulva and, as the abdomen is accessible, bimanual examination of the pelvic organs. It does not, however, allow adequate demonstration of genital prolapse or inspection of the vaginal walls. Some patients find this position particularly exposing — if you partially cover the thighs and knees they may feel less embarrassed. The dorsal position is sometimes mistakenly called the 'lithotomy' position. **10**
2. In the ***left-lateral position*** the patient lies on her left side with her arms in front of her and her hips flexed. This position allows adequate inspection of the perineum, anus and posterior vulval area. It also allows good inspection of the vaginal walls and demonstration of prolapse. As the abdomen is not fully accessible in this position, bimanual examination is not adequate. **10**
3. The ***Sims' position*** is the best position for inspecting the anterior vaginal wall: when the introitus is opened with the aid of a Sims' speculum the vagina fills out with air. In this position the patient brings her buttocks to the edge of the bed, her left arm is placed behind her back and her thighs are flexed (the upper one more than the lower). Again, the abdomen is not fully accessible and bimanual examination is inadequate. **10**

Total mark out of 30: divide by 3 for final mark

STATION 10.4

Complications of termination of pregnancy (TOP)

Marks

Candidate's instructions

Discuss with the examiner the short-term and long-term complications of termination of pregnancy.

Examiner's instructions

The following points should be discussed and marked as shown:

- *Rate of haemorrhage necessitating blood transfusion* is around 1.5/1000. Lower for early procedures (1.2/1000 at <13 weeks; 8.5/1000 at >20 weeks). **2**
- *Uterine perforation* at the time of surgical TOP occurs in 1–4/1000. Lower incidence if performed early in pregnancy and by an experienced clinician. **2**
- *Cervical trauma*: the rate of damage to the external cervical os at the time of surgical abortion is 1%. The rate is lower when abortions are performed early in pregnancy and when they are performed by experienced clinicians. **2**
- *Failed abortion/continuation of pregnancy*: this is a complication of first-trimester abortion. The rate for surgical abortion is around 2.3/1000; for medical abortion the rate is around 6/1000 **4**
- *Post-abortion infection*: genital tract infection of varying degrees of severity, including pelvic inflammatory disease, occurs in up to 10% of cases. The risk is reduced when prophylactic antibiotics are given or when lower genital tract infection has been excluded by screening. **4**
- *Future reproductive outcome*: there are no proven associations between induced abortion and subsequent infertility or preterm labour. **2**
- *Psychological sequelae*: only a small minority of women experience any long-term adverse psychological sequelae after abortion. Early distress, although common, is usually a continuation of symptoms present before the abortion. Conversely, long-lasting, negative effects on both mothers and their children are reported where abortion has been denied. **4**

Total mark out of 20: divide by 2 for final mark

STATION 10.5	
Counselling for molar pregnancy	Marks

Candidate's instructions

You are asked to see a 26-year-old secretary who has been referred with a threatened miscarriage. Discuss with the examiner what you would do and how you would counsel the patient.

Examiner's instructions

The following assessment and procedures should be discussed by the candidate:

	Marks
• History should include questions about how many weeks pregnant, planned pregnancy, how much bleeding and pain (which started first?), passage of any products.	**2**
• Assess risk factors for ectopic pregnancy: PID, type of contraception, previous ectopic.	**2**
• Examination for abdominal tenderness, VE — os open or closed, adnexal tenderness.	**2**
• Arrange ultrasound scan, blood tests, group and save (note Rh factor), FBC; note possible need for HCG quantification if worried about ectopic.	**2**
• Sympathetic explanation.	**2**

The candidate is told that the ultrasound scan suggests a hydropic pregnancy with no fetus identified. What is the likely diagnosis and how would you manage it?

	Marks
• Molar pregnancy (complete mole).	**2**
• Needs HCG measurement.	**1**
• Evacuation of uterus — explain risks of bleeding and damage to the uterus.	**1**
• IV access and crossmatch blood.	**1**
• Evacuation by senior doctor.	**2**
• Follow-up includes serial HCGs (blood/urine), registration with centre, contraceptive advice and advice about future pregnancies. Reason for follow-up — risk of recurrence.	**2**
• Counselling should include assurance of good prognosis.	**1**

Total mark out of 20: divide by 2 for final mark

STATION 10.6

Labour ward priorities — preparatory station

Candidate's instructions

You are the labour ward registrar taking over at 8.30 a.m. You have an SHO who has done 3 months of obstetrics, a sister in charge who is very experienced, and the anaesthetic registrar.

The labour ward board looks as follows:

Labour Ward				
Room	**Name**	**Parity**	**Gestation**	**Comments**
1	Adams	1	39/40	Elective caesarean section
2	Bethell	0	36/40	?Early labour; ?breech
3	Campbell	4	40+/40	Del. 7.00; placenta not del. 500 ml blood loss
4	Devine	2	42+/40	Cervix closed; IOL; post-dates; decels
5	Evans	0	34/40	?SROM; twins
6	Ferdinand	0	40/40	Fully dilated, 6.00, pushing
7	Goodison	1	41/40	Del. 6.30; second degree tear
8	Harrison	1	39/40	5 cm at 6.00; (2 cm at 2.00, 5 cm at 10.00 Syntocinon); meconium/decels

Discuss with the examiner at the next station which women would be your priorities and how you would manage the patients.

STATION 10.7

Labour ward priorities — examination station

Marks

Examiner's instructions

The following points should be discussed and marks awarded as shown:

1. ***Priorities:*** **6**

 - *Room 3*: Risk of postpartum haemorrhage. You will need to look briefly at her to assess loss and you could ask the SHO to put a line in, crossmatch blood, and prepare for theatre.
 - *Room 4*: This trace needs urgent review and a decision on whether to continue with the induction or to deliver.
 - *Room 8*: This lady also needs reviewing as she has a secondary arrest and possibly fetal distress.

2. ***Management:*** **8**

 - *Room 1*: Can be deferred, not an emergency and other work must take priority.
 - *Room 2*: Midwifery case initially. She may need a scan if the midwife cannot determine presentation on vaginal examination, which the SHO may be able to do. Not an immediate priority.
 - *Room 3*: Potential problem. May need immediate action as she has a postpartum haemorrhage. This may mean a manual removal but she needs resuscitation and sorting out for theatre. May need further Syntocinon or ergometrine (if no contraindication) prior to theatre. Check that she has been catheterized. The SHO can sort much of this out and prepare her for theatre.
 - *Room 4*: Trace needs urgent review. If the decelerations are significant, she may need immediate delivery or consider tocolysis to gain time. A vaginal examination is important — she may be progressing as she is a multip.
 - *Room 5*: Not an immediate priority. She does need a speculum exam. and possibly a VE, which the SHO can do. Will need to review at some point but not now.
 - *Room 6*: Possibly needs delivering in the near future. You need to know more details. May have had a long passive stage. What is the CTG like? If the CTG is O.K., may not be an immediate problem — labour ward sister may need to help the midwife looking after this woman.

- *Room 7*: Needs suturing but this does not necessarily need a doctor. Concern needs to be raised that she has delivered 2 hours previously and may have bled significantly.
- *Room 8*: This room needs reviewing — it may be necessary to stop the Syntocinon whilst sorting out Room 4 and possibly Room 3.

3. ***Other considerations:*** 6

- *Room 1*: May need to call for help and ask the consultant to help.
- *Room 2*: Ensure good communication, liaising with anaesthetist and paediatricians.
- *Room 3*: Alert theatre staff as two women may need to be delivered at the same time — may need to get a second theatre.

Total mark out of 20: divide by 2 for final mark

STATION 10.8

Fetal anomaly

Marks

Candidate's instructions

Mrs Jones is a 30-year-old woman who is 20 weeks pregnant in her second pregnancy. This is an IVF pregnancy. She had primary infertility and had a termination of her first IVF pregnancy because of Edwards' syndrome. In this pregnancy she had an ultrasound scan at 12 weeks that showed a fetal nuchal thickness which equates with a 1:5000 risk of Down's syndrome (according to local protocols). She has just had her mid-trimester ultrasound scan and the ultrasonographer has found choroid plexus cysts (CPC).

You have been called to see her. Explain to the examiner how you would counsel her and what follow-up you would arrange.

Examiner's instructions

The following points should be discussed and marked as indicated:

- Explain that CPCs are a 'soft' marker associated with chromosomal abnormalities. The finding on its own is usually benign. (Risk of Down's syndrome with isolated CPCs increases by a factor of 5 against the background risk — in her case, from 1:5000 to 1:1000. You would not therefore automatically need an amniocentesis). **4**
- Ask about other markers on the scan. Features associated with Edwards' syndrome (trisomy 18) are: agenesis of corpus callosum, posterior fossa abnormalities, micrognathia, low-set ears, hypertelorism, clenched hand with overlapping index finger, club foot, rocker-bottom foot, renal anomalies, omphalocele, diaphragmatic hernia, heart defects, single umbilical artery, polyhydramnios and raised nuchal thickness. **4**
- Down's syndrome is associated with ventriculomegaly, brachycephaly, flat facies, small ears, heart defects, hyperechogenic bowel, duodenal atresia, clinodactyly, short humerus, short femur, sandal foot. **4**
- In the absence of other markers, and with the reassuring nuchal thickness, you can discuss the options reassuringly. CPCs are found in 1–2% of normal pregnancies. Risk of aneuploidy with isolated CPCs 1–4%. **3**

- Options are to wait and see if the cysts resolve (as they often do) or to consider karyotyping in view of the previous Edwards' baby. Risk of amniocentesis approximately 1%. This is obviously a difficult decision, given the history of IVF and previous termination. 3
- Consider referral to a Fetal Medicine Unit. 2

Total mark out of 20: divide by 2 for final mark

STATION 10.9

Perinatal mortality: definitions

Marks

Candidate's instructions

Discuss with the examiner the definitions of the following terms: livebirth, stillbirth, stillbirth rate, early neonatal mortality rate, late neonatal mortality rate, infant mortality rate and perinatal mortality rate.

Examiner's instructions

- *Livebirth:* the complete expulsion or extraction from its mother of a baby, irrespective of gestational age, which then shows any signs of life such as breathing, beating of the heart, pulsation of the umbilical cord, or definite movement of voluntary muscles. **4**
- *Stillbirth:* birth of a baby, from 24 completed weeks of gestation, who shows no signs of life after birth. This is the UK definition. The international definition only includes babies from 28 completed weeks. **4**
- *Stillbirth rate:* the number of stillbirths per 1000 *total* births (stillbirths and livebirths). **2**
- *Early neonatal mortality rate*: the number of liveborn babies dying within the first week of life (early neonatal period) per 1000 livebirths. **2**
- *Late neonatal mortality rate*: the number of liveborn babies dying from the end of the first week of life until the end of the fourth week (late neonatal period) per 1000 livebirths. **2**
- *Infant mortality rate*: the number of liveborn babies dying within the first year of life (infant period) per 1000 livebirths. **2**
- *Perinatal mortality rate*: the number of stillbirths and first-week deaths (i.e. stillbirths and early neonatal deaths) per 1000 total births (stillbirths and livebirths). **4**

Total mark out of 20: divide by 2 for final mark

STATION 10.10

Audit of urinary catheter

Marks

Candidate's instructions

Three years ago at Obgyn District General Hospital it was noted that women who had a Foley catheter inserted into the bladder at total abdominal hysterectomy and left on free drainage for 48 hours had fewer postoperative urinary tract infections than those where the bladder was catheterized and emptied just prior to surgery and the catheter removed ('in and out' catheterization).

This led to the writing of a protocol for preoperative catheterization which was agreed by all consultant gynaecologists:

Protocol for bladder catheterization prior to total abdominal hysterectomy

Following induction of anaesthesia and transfer of the patient to the operating table, a 12FG Foley catheter is to be inserted into the bladder, using an aseptic technique. The catheter is then to be connected to a sterile, closed bag and left on continuous drainage for 48 hours.

Discuss with the examiner how you would design an audit to ascertain how well this protocol is being adhered to and what steps you would take if the audit reveals lapses in compliance. (You are not being asked to comment on or criticize the protocol.)

Examiner's instruction

The following should be discussed, and marks allocated as indicated:

1. ***The key components of an audit:*** 5
   - Find the patients who should have been managed by this protocol in the given time period.
   - Would a percentage sample be sufficient?

- Determine a method of establishing whether the protocol was followed for each patient.
- Ascertain the outcome.
- Analyse the data, including quantification of missing data.
- Consider sampling bias.
- Identify why the protocol was not followed in some cases.

2. ***Feedback of results to departmental staff:*** **5**
   - Should be done sensitively.
   - Consider confidentiality.
   - What reactions might be expected?
3. ***Considerations if organizational changes are needed to facilitate/improve compliance:*** **5**
   - Resource implications.
   - Ways to achieve consistent implementation.
4. ***Considerations if any elements of the protocol require modification:*** **5**
   - Recent research data/College guidelines.
   - Has there been criticism of protocol by user groups?
5. ***Decision on when audit should be repeated:*** **5**
   - How long will it take for organizational/protocol changes to be implemented?
   - If the protocol is changed a second audit may not be comparable.

Total mark out of 25: divide by 5 and then multiply by 2 for final mark

INDEX